WHEN CHILDREN FEEL PAIN

When Children Feel Pain

From Everyday Aches to Chronic Conditions

**Rachel Rabkin Peachman
and Anna C. Wilson**

Harvard University Press

Cambridge, Massachusetts, & London, England   2022

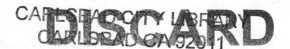

Library of Congress Cataloging-in-Publication Data
Names: Peachman, Rachel Rabkin, author. | Wilson, Anna C., author.
Title: When children feel pain : from everyday aches to chronic conditions /
Rachel Rabkin Peachman and Anna C. Wilson.
Description: Cambridge, Massachusetts : Harvard University Press, 2022. |
Includes bibliographical references and index.
Identifiers: LCCN 2022001785 | ISBN 9780674185029 (cloth)
Subjects: LCSH: Pain in children. | Pain—Treatment. | Pain—Psychological aspects.
Classification: LCC RJ365 .P42 2022 | DDC 618.92/0472—dc23/eng/20220223
LC record available at https://lccn.loc.gov/2022001785

To my parents, Elizabeth and Eric Rabkin
—*Rachel*

To my parents, Philip and Mary Long
—*Anna*

Contents

Authors' Note

Unless otherwise noted in the endnotes, direct quotes in this book are taken from our own interviews and conversations with researchers and families. Quotes pulled from other published works or public talks are referenced as such.

To protect the privacy of the children and parents, we use only their first names in most instances, and in some cases use pseudonyms. If a full name is given, that is the person's actual name.

We are eternally grateful to the numerous scientists, clinicians, and families who shared their knowledge and experiences with us as we worked on this book. Not every individual who spoke with us is directly mentioned within these pages, but each influenced our thinking and we could not have produced this work without them. We thank them all wholeheartedly for their generosity, time, and insights.

WHEN CHILDREN FEEL PAIN

Introduction
Beyond Boo-Boos

The long-term payoffs of addressing short-term pain

A six-month-old is lying on his back on an exam table in a pediatrician's office. "There, there," says the nurse, "this will only sting for a second!" The baby boy reaches out for his mother, on the other side of the room, and shrieks when the nurse injects a vaccination into his thigh.

A five-year-old complains of a stomachache before school one morning. Her mother pats her on the back and says, "I'm sorry you're not feeling well, but we're going to be late. Let's get moving!"

A ten-year-old and her father leave the orthopedist after a long day in the emergency department. She has a brand-new cast on one arm but walks out with no instructions on how to manage the throbbing ache she feels.

A fourteen-year-old girl tells her pediatrician that she has been having headaches after school at least twice a week. "That's probably just stress-related," he says as he peers into her ear canal. "How are your classes going?"

An eighteen-year-old stumbles on the soccer field and clutches his ankle. "Walk it off," yells his coach. "Get back out there!"

At first glance, these episodes don't seem to warrant a whole lot of concern. Kids get hurt and experience pain all the time, and they usually recover just fine, right? A sympathetic pat on the back, a well-meaning shout of encouragement, or a Band-Aid often does the trick. But how would you know if you had truly addressed the problem? What effect do painful experiences—whether a little needle poke or a major break—have on a child?

Many adults have no idea. In fact, most people—including many parents, doctors, and psychologists—do not realize what pain can do to a child's developing nervous system in the short term or the long term. Few are aware that many children experience recurrent or chronic pain that can severely disrupt their lives and continue into adulthood.

The vignettes above are typical examples of how children's pain is often dismissed, minimized, and flat-out ignored. Those instances are not anomalies. Episodes of under-recognized pain in children unfold across the country, every day, in homes, medical settings, and playgrounds, among other places. This is not because of a lack of love for these children. It may not even be because there is a lack of access to medical care (though sometimes that is a factor). It is because pain—especially pain in children—is poorly understood. And when pain is misunderstood, it gets sidelined and mismanaged, and can cause far-reaching and lasting damage.

We'd like to change that. Anna (a pediatric pain psychologist) and Rachel (a health and science journalist with a personal history of chronic pain) joined forces on this book to make clear that children's early experiences with pain matter deeply and can shape future perception of pain and overall development. But our message is not one of doom and gloom. On the contrary, we will demonstrate that adults can do so much more—for the children in their lives and even for themselves—than sit idly by. Whether you are a parent, a grandparent, a medical professional, a teacher, or anyone else who cares for children, you have the opportunity to affect how children respond to and cope with pain, and your influence now can help them throughout their lives. This book will give you the tools to do so and point you to resources that will make managing children's pain a priority. The first step is to acknowledge the need for better pain management. The next steps will become clear as you read further, and we hope you will be inspired to take them.

The Neglected Sufferers of the Pain Epidemic

In recent years, the medical community, policy makers, and news media have begun to acknowledge and address the severity of our country's adult pain epidemic. By the latest estimates, some seventy million American adults endure chronic pain (generally defined as pain that persists for more than twelve weeks), which means it affects more people than diabetes, heart disease, and cancer combined. In addition to the enormous physical and emotional suffering that chronic pain causes, it costs the United States over $500 billion dollars in lost productivity and medical treatments each year.[1] It has also helped to fuel a widespread dependence on pain-relieving opioid medications, which are tied to an estimated 130 overdose deaths each day.[2] But adults are not the only ones suffering. An estimated five percent of children in the United States experience moderate to severe chronic pain, annually costing about $19.5 billion.[3]

Rachel knows that suffering all too well. After being diagnosed with scoliosis at age eight, and wearing a back brace from ages eight through sixteen, she later developed increasingly unbearable backaches, muscle spasms, and pinched nerves as a young adult. Rachel is no stranger to the ways pain can infiltrate your being, one stealthy attack at a time. She also knows the frustration of searching for decades for help from physicians, physical therapists, and all manner of holistic healers, and finding little or no relief. It is a hopeless place to be—and too many people have been there.

Why is it so hard for patients to find appropriate help for their pain? For starters, the medical professionals on the front lines—internists, family physicians, and surgeons—have little training in pain management. Unless they specialize in pain, most medical students receive a mere one to six hours of education in pain management. Veterinary school students are required to have significantly more education in how to alleviate pain in animals than would-be physicians are required to have in treating pain in humans.[4] For many clinicians, then, pain management translates into prescribing pain relievers, such as opioids, which are often ineffective in the long term and are notoriously addictive. But thanks to the efforts of researchers, professional societies (such as the International Association for the Study of Pain and the American Academy of Pain Medicine), patient advocacy groups (such as the American Chronic Pain Association and the US Pain Foundation), and national agencies (such as the Centers for Disease Control and Prevention and the National Institutes of Health), we are slowly starting to recognize the need for better pain management in adults that extends beyond medication. In 2015, government agencies, led by the National Institutes of Health and the Department of Health and Human Services, unveiled the National Pain Strategy, which defines chronic pain as a disease in its own right and provides a comprehensive approach for addressing it in adults—an important acknowledgment of an issue that has been neglected for too long.

For children, however, the situation remains dismal. Specifically, in the United States, Canada, and Western European countries, there is an astonishing lack of awareness among members of the public, physicians, and even parents regarding our smallest sufferers. For instance, although the National Pain Strategy calls out the importance of preventing the development of chronic pain, children's pain is not even mentioned in the plan. This is despite decades of research showing that pediatric pain is prevalent, disabling, and costly, and that having chronic pain in childhood is a risk factor for chronic pain in adulthood.

Pediatric pain is overlooked on not only a national level but an individual level. Multiple studies published over two decades in premier journals show one in five children suffering chronic pain, but only a small fraction of them receiving treatments that may help them.[5] This is not for lack of treatment options. There are numerous scientifically proven therapies for managing pain in children. Yet, according to research published in the *Clinical Journal of Pain,* even when children with chronic pain are referred for specialized pain treatments, such as pain psychology or physical therapy, fewer than half receive these services. This is possibly due to the limited number of pediatric pain specialists available and limited healthcare coverage for these therapies (for both children and adults), among other barriers.[6]

Strikingly, research has also found disparate treatment of adults versus children suffering the same conditions or undergoing the same procedures: historically, adults receive at least two times the pain medication doses that children do.[7] And the younger the child, the less pain control is likely to be provided. "A seventeen-year-old teenager is going to get better pain control than a seventeen-month-old toddler, who's going to get better pain control than a seventeen-day-old infant with the same underlying condition," says Stefan Friedrichsdorf, medical director of pediatric pain medicine and palliative care at the University of California San Francisco Benioff

Children's Hospital. "Pain management in the United States and Western countries is still abysmal."

There are many reasons that pain control in children has been a low priority. Chapter 2 examines why in depth, but briefly, it is important to note here that it has taken decades for medical professionals even to acknowledge that children feel pain as intensely as adults do. As recently as the 1980s, babies were undergoing invasive medical procedures, such as open-heart surgery, without anesthesia or analgesics because physicians believed that infants' nervous systems were not mature enough to feel the pain. While ample scientific research has proven that assumption to be categorically false, old habits die hard, and managing a child's pain is all too often an afterthought for physicians focused on dealing with the ailment at hand. Even in cases where medical professionals are aware that pain control is needed, they are frequently hesitant to give strong pain medications to children for fear of dangerous side effects, damage to developing brains, and worries about opioid addiction. (Research has found these fears to be largely unwarranted when it comes to children, as discussed in later chapters.) In those instances where pain control ends up being subpar, many physicians have rationalized this shortcoming by telling themselves that babies and children won't ultimately remember the pain later on.

Evidence shows, however, that while babies and children may not consciously remember painful experiences, their nervous systems certainly will. Research dating back more than twenty years has found that early exposures to pain—and early responses to those episodes by clinicians and parents—can shape a child's neural pathways.

One of the most important studies on pain in infancy was published in the medical journal *The Lancet* in 1997.[8] The researchers evaluated infants in three categories: baby boys who had undergone circumcision without receiving pain management; baby boys who had been circumcised in conjunction with a topical pain treatment; and baby boys who had not been circumcised. These infants were videotaped during routine vaccinations at four and six months old to assess their response to brief needle pain. Researchers who were not privy to the backgrounds of the infants then watched the videotapes and rated their pain responses based on facial expressions and how long they cried. They found that infants who had not been circumcised cried least after getting their shots. The infants who cried most were those who had been circumcised without proper pain management. The finding implies that infants can indeed develop memories related to pain (which may be subconscious but are memories nonetheless) and these memories influence how they later experience pain. The study also shows that when painful procedures are inadequately managed, an infant's nervous system can become more sensitized with each subsequent exposure to pain. Every painful experience builds on the last.

Numerous other studies, particularly those involving babies in neonatal intensive care units, have found that poorly managed pain early in life can actually change the wiring in the brain and have lasting physiological impact—which has the potential not only to make children more sensitive to pain episodes but also to increase their risk of developing chronic pain. Once a child develops chronic pain, it can turn into a life sentence. Up to two-thirds of children who experience episodes of chronic pain go on to have chronic pain as adults. Alarmingly, for some of these chronic sufferers, their painful experiences began early, often in healthcare settings. This means that improving pain treatment in pediatric medical settings may be critical to reducing the incidence of chronic pain in adults.

The tragic consequence, then, of undertreating children in pain is not limited to the discomfort they feel in a particular moment but extends to lasting harm as this experience affects their developing neuropathways. In other words, that boo-boo you may dismiss as inconsequential has the potential to be so much more.

Pioneering Pediatric Pain Centers

Fortunately, there are pain researchers and clinicians who know how to treat pediatric pain, and they've developed the strategies to do it. Over the past twenty to thirty years, these experts have dedicated their careers to furthering our understanding of pain in children. They are a relatively small group, but working diligently to improve on the status quo. Among them is one of us—Anna, who works at the Pediatric Pain Management and Coping Clinics at Oregon Health and Science University in Portland, Oregon. To come up with solutions, she spends her days counseling children with chronic pain and researching the effects that pain has on families. Anna has witnessed up close how proper pain management can transform the lives of children and their parents. Sadly, gaining access to these solutions takes far too long for most families.

Take the case of Taylor and her ill-fated roller-skating session. At almost nine years old, she was in gym class in her Wisconsin school when she lost her balance and fell to the floor. The accident might have been of no consequence had it not been for the fact that another student skating nearby then tumbled over her. The searing pain in Taylor's left foot was instant. But the diagnosis of the injury took much longer.

Taylor, a thoughtful girl with an easy smile, was promptly forced to stop playing basketball and taking dance lessons. "I couldn't walk or play outside or do anything," she recalls. Her mother, Jodi, says their family doctor "first told us to give it some time" and prescribed rest and a bandage, and then physical therapy, yet the pain was unrelenting.

In the months that followed, Taylor underwent X-rays, MRIs, a CT scan, and blood tests, none of which revealed evidence of a break, sprain, or other clear injury. Her primary symptom was pain—so severe that she could not put pressure on her foot, let alone walk or run. At school, she used crutches to get around, and at home she resorted to crawling, hopping on one foot, or piggyback rides from her older brother to get where she needed to go.

Her mother was desperate to help, but none of the medical professionals she consulted could grasp what was going on. "I didn't know what to do," Jodi remembers. "Watching Taylor struggle, especially for so long, was heartbreaking. If I could have switched places with her, I would have."

After a torturous year and a half, Taylor's orthopedist finally suggested she see Dr. Friedrichsdorf, who was then the medical director of pain medicine and palliative care at Children's Hospitals and Clinics of Minnesota—a manageable driving distance from Taylor's home. He and his team immediately recognized Taylor's condition as complex regional pain syndrome, which is a misfiring within the peripheral and central nervous systems that causes pain signals to go into overdrive and stay turned on even after an initial injury or trauma has healed.

Dr. Friedrichsdorf came up with a treatment plan for Taylor that included physical therapy, stress-reduction strategies, topical pain-relief patches, and a focus on returning to her normal life and sleep routine, among other things. (For more on these techniques, see Chapter 12.) "That turned things around so fast," Taylor's mother says, that "if I didn't see it myself, I wouldn't have believed it." She recalls thinking, "*finally,* someone understands what this is, has experience with it, and knows how to fix it!"

Someone understands. It is what every child in pain hopes to find: a doctor, or at least a parent, who gets it, doesn't discount it, and can offer real support. Compared to most children affected by chronic pain, Taylor was lucky. She found a knowledgeable practitioner at the forefront of pain management close enough to her home, and her family had the resources to benefit from his help. But experienced pain specialists are few and far between. There is a gaping hole within the field of pain management that makes it extremely difficult for children to gain access to medical centers that offer effective treatments led by practitioners with the appropriate knowledge. Some children who endure chronic pain never find anyone who understands.

The Promise of a Better Future

But imagine, for a moment, that we could alter this story line. Imagine flipping the pages of this narrative back to the beginning, all the way to when children have their earliest experiences with pain. Maybe it's the day a baby is born and a nurse draws blood from his heel to test for congenital conditions. Or perhaps it's when a preschooler falls against a coffee table and needs stitches to her head. Or it could be when a teenager starts to develop a nagging backache after a sports injury. What if we could learn to spot that pain better, acknowledge it, and treat it before those developing neurons get out of control?

Research tells us that we can. We have the power to alter this trajectory. We do not need to settle for poor pain management in children and the resulting increased risk of chronic pain in adult-hood. Contrary to previous thinking, studies show that the effective use of pain medication, even opioids, in children does *not* hinder brain development or lead to addiction when monitored by experienced physicians. What's more, medication is just one of many options. A host of interventions, such as cognitive behavioral therapy, physical therapy, meditation, and acupuncture, can be employed to prevent and treat pain—and guard against chronic pain before it starts. There is no reason for children to suffer. They will be healthier, happier, and more functional people if they receive the pain therapies they sorely need.

To be clear, this declaration doesn't apply only to children dealing with the aftermath of major accidents and medical traumas. Interventions that prevent or reduce pain should be used even during seemingly minor procedures, such as vaccinations. Every needle poke, sprain, and pain-causing illness is an opportunity to influence for the better a child's pain responses, coping mechanisms, and relationship with healthcare professionals.

If this seems like a daunting directive, relax. Some of the best-proven tools to reduce children's pain are risk-free, noninvasive, and consistent with most parents' natural instincts. Strategies that have been shown to alleviate discomfort and anxiety include letting caregivers hold their children during medical procedures; allowing babies to breastfeed or swallow a sweet solution during vaccinations (and giving older kids lollipops); and distracting children before a surgery with songs, breathing exercises, or iPads.

Another bonus: these tactics illustrate that parents and other caregivers can play a major role in alleviating children's discomfort and advocating for appropriate treatments. But so far, little of this information has made its way into most parenting books, clinicians' offices, or even medical school curriculums. In the majority of cases, children still go undertreated, despite what we know could help them, whether they're undergoing minor medical procedures or dealing with severe diseases.

Christine Chambers, professor of pediatrics, psychology, neuroscience, and pain management at Dalhousie University in Halifax, Nova Scotia, is acutely aware of this disconnect. "When you look at all the different areas where children experience pain today—in the neonatal intensive care unit or surgery, vaccination pain, pain associated with disease, and pain in the emergency department—there are still 'knowledge to action gaps,' as we call them, where we have a lot of science to tell us what we could be doing and should be doing. Yet what is happening for kids every day is not consistent with the evidence," she explains. When Dr. Chambers discusses the issue with parents, she's found that many are shocked to learn their child's pain *could* be alleviated, and yet it is not. "They all say, 'How come I didn't know about this? I assumed that if there was something that could be done to lessen my child's pain, it would be offered.'"

The reason for the gaps, says Dr. Chambers, is that scientific research and policies based on it can take up to seventeen years to get implemented in practice, and only fourteen percent of research ever makes its way into doctor's offices.[9] Do we really want to wait seventeen years to implement strategies that pain researchers have proven can stop children from suffering from the short-term sting of a shot or the drawn-out pain of a long-term illness?

Parents cannot stand to wait. Our children cannot stand to wait. This body of research exists now and is only growing more robust as time goes on. It can be put into practice today, especially if parents advocate for it. It's time to bridge the gap between what we know about pediatric pain management and how much is actually implemented and accessible. Pain treatment for children must be a priority.

To all the parents who have picked up this book: You will see that this is not a parenting book per se, but we hope it will profoundly affect how you raise your children.

To all the medical professionals who are reading this book: It is not meant to be a textbook, but we sincerely hope you will take this information into your medical school classes, pediatric exam rooms, operating rooms, and emergency departments, and put it into practice with the young patients you treat.

To all the adults who have endured pain or are burdened by chronic pain now and are seeking insight in this book: Keep reading. It is not too late to affect your experience or the experience of your children. Though this is not a self-help book, the research found herein will offer a deeper understanding of your own pain and how it may affect your family—and show you possible paths toward relief.

To any who have found their way to this book perhaps without realizing why it might be relevant: This is for you, too. This is a book about the universal human experience of pain, and how our bodies learn to react to pain from the first moment our nervous systems take form. Our great hope is that, whether you have children, treat children, or have suffered your own episodes of pain and discomfort, you will embrace the notion that we have the ability to act. Solving our nation's chronic pain epidemic starts with acknowledging pain and responding to it appropriately. If we give pain the attention it deserves early in life, we can minimize short-term suffering, and halt the development of long-term chronic pain in the next generation.

Chapter 1

How and Why Do We Feel Pain?

Demystifying the neurobiology of this fiery signal

Pain is always real, no matter what is causing it.
—*Lorimer Moseley, pain researcher at the*
University of South Australia

How is it that pain, one of our most primal experiences, can be invisible yet unmistakably present? Indescribable yet undeniable? Intangible yet concrete? Subjective yet universal?

Understanding pain has been a pursuit filled with contradictions for centuries. But for most of modern medical history scientists believed that pain was a purely biomechanical phenomenon. The belief, popularized by the seventeenth-century philosopher René Descartes, was that, when the body gets injured, a signal is sent from the injured area through a physical pathway to the brain, where it registers a degree of pain that is proportional to the injury. The mind, Descartes proposed, was entirely separate from the body and therefore had nothing to do with physical pain. Over the course of many years and many iterations of pain theories, however, we've learned that the perception of somatic pain (which is of the body) is inextricably tied not only to the brain but also to the psychological workings of the mind.[1]

What we feel, and how much we hurt, is dependent on the brain's interpretation of a physical sensation *and* on the brain's assessment of a multitude of psychological and contextual factors, including the circumstances of the pain, a person's previous experiences with pain, and emotions such as stress or fear.

The official definition of pain, first put forth in 1979 by the International Association for the Study of Pain and updated in 2020, makes clear that pain is simultaneously physical (sensory) and psychological (emotional). The definition states, in part, that pain is: "an unpleasant sensory and emotional experience associated with, or resembling that associated with, actual or potential tissue damage." The definition also offers six key points for critical context:

- Pain is always a personal experience that is influenced to varying degrees by biological, psychological, and social factors.
- Pain and nociception (the nervous system's encoding of harmful stimuli) are different phenomena. Pain cannot be inferred solely from activity in sensory neurons.
- Through their life experiences, individuals learn the concept of pain.
- A person's report of an experience as pain should be respected.
- Although pain usually serves an adaptive role, it may have adverse effects on function and social and psychological well-being.[2]

In other words, physical pain is an experience of both the body and mind and there is no such thing as a one-size-fits-all pain signal. When you stub your toe, for instance, you might perceive a drastically different pain level than someone next to you who experiences the exact same injury. Your brain bases its response to the sensation on the information it has previously gathered in your life, in your body, and no one else's. So while we tend to think of pain as a universal experience, how we perceive it as extremely individual and situational.

Fortunately for us, because our perception of pain is influenced by psychological and contextual factors (such as our experiences, our memories, our environment, and our anxiety level), we can use psychological and behavioral strategies to moderate our pain signals and dial down how much we hurt. We have the power to change how we feel pain. To act on this possibility, first it's important to understand the difference between the two broad forms of pain: acute pain and chronic pain.

Acute Pain

Acute pain is generally the type of pain you feel when you break your leg, get an infection, or touch a hot stove. Though it doesn't feel good, its purpose is to protect you from further harm. The reason we have that "unpleasant sensory and emotional experience" is to warn us that our body is in danger and we should stop what we're doing and take action to address the pain. If this pain alarm system didn't go off, we might not be alerted to the fact that anything required fixing, and we'd likely get increasingly injured and sick. Acute pain, then, is typically protective and short-term, and tends to go away when the injury or illness resolves.

How, exactly, does the body and brain clue us in to what we're feeling? We process sensory information through our central nervous system (which includes the brain and the spinal cord) and our peripheral nervous system (which includes all the nerves that branch out from the brain and spinal cord and extend to our muscles and even our organs). In general, it works like this: if you place your hand on the burner of a hot stove, pain receptors (peripheral nerve endings called nociceptors) in the hand perceive the painful sensation and release rapid-fire nerve signals (in the form of chemical messengers called neurotransmitters) through an ascending pathway (going up) to the spinal cord.

At the back of the spinal cord, the dorsal horn receives the chemical signals at a checkpoint that you might imagine as a set of gates. Based on the information received there, the gates may open wide and send the sensory messages flooding through to the brain, or they may close and limit the sensory messages that reach the brain. This concept, known as the gate control theory, revolutionized much of our understanding of pain when it was proposed in 1965 by British neurophysiologist Patrick David Wall, and Canadian psychologist Ronald Melzack. The theory contends that both physical and psychological factors can open or close the gates and influence which messages the brain receives. Factors that keep the gates open and send pain messages through to the brain include stress, fear, and focusing on the injury or site of the pain. Factors that can close the gates include being relaxed, perceiving an additional, non-painful sensation, and focusing on an unrelated task separate from the pain.[3] The gate control theory explains why soldiers with severe wounds may feel no pain while they're in the thick of a battle. When they're absorbed in the fight, their bodies are in a highly aroused physiological state, which can temporarily inhibit the ability of the nerve cells in the dorsal horn to send pain signals. In that state, the gate is closed. It's as if the body is saying, "there are other important things happening right now, and there's no room to process pain signals." The gate control theory also explains why holding someone's hand while getting a vaccine injection, or petting your cat while recovering from a fall, or even rubbing the area around an injury can lessen the perception of pain. All of those additional sensory inputs take up space in the pain-signaling pathway, leaving less room for the pain signals to make their way through to the brain.[4]

When chemical messages do move past the "gates" of the spinal cord, they go up through the spinothalamic tract (the ascending pain pathway) to the thalamus within the brain. Known as the brain's relay station, the thalamus receives the messages and sends them to the cerebral cortex to make sense of the situation while taking into account signals and cues from multiple systems such as the sensory, visual, and motor systems.

To paraphrase Lorimer Moseley, a pain researcher and professor of neuroscience at the University of South Australia, if your brain could talk through its thought process at that point, the thalamus might say, "Hey! Something dangerous has touched my hand!" It would then send that message to the cortex, which would ask itself, "What happened? Should I stop what I'm doing? How much should this hurt?" In the case of a hand on a hot stove burner, the cortex would likely decide, "This is a serious situation that could damage my hand unless I move quickly, so I'm going to make this hurt a lot!" Once the brain has arrived at a conclusion (a process that takes a split second), it sends descending messages back down through the spinal cord (the descending pain pathway) and peripheral nervous system and those messages inform how your body responds to the threat and how much pain you feel.[5]

It's important to note that, as this process is happening, messages also pass through a number of areas of the brain that control autonomic functions, such as heart rate, breathing, perspiration, and the release of certain hormones that act as neurotransmitters. These include serotonin and dopamine (commonly known as feel-good chemicals, which can dampen pain signals), and adrenaline and epinephrine (which can rev up your body in preparation for a threat).

These autonomic processes explain why we may respond to pain with a racing heart, shallow breaths, and a cold sweat. Like acute pain itself, this stress response, called the "fight or flight" response, is meant to alert us that we need to act or get away from the painful sensation.

Ultimately, says Dr. Moseley, how much pain you feel depends on the brain's evaluation of this question: "How dangerous is this *really*?" While the answer may seem evident in the instance of a hand on a hot stove, your perception of pain may vary widely depending on your emotions, beliefs, previous experiences, and the context of the sensation.[6]

For example, if you're a consummate baker who's gotten used to the occasional burn, and you're having fun making cookies with your kids on a relaxing Sunday afternoon, an inadvertent burn on your hand may not even slow you down. You've learned from past experiences that the pain is temporary and that the wound will heal quickly. You don't get anxious about the injury, and when your brain evaluates the context of the pain, your attitude, and your memories, it will interpret the threat as minor, and send descending messages to the hand that signal a low level of pain.

If, however, you're a child who is new to cooking, alone in the kitchen, and feeling anxious about using the stove without permission, a burn on your hand may stop you in your tracks. Your brain has never experienced this particular sensation before, so it can't rely on memory, and as it takes in the stress and fear building within you it interprets the threat as an emergency. The brain then sends descending messages back through the spinal cord and peripheral nervous system that will likely crank up the pain.

This experience may then go on to inform how much pain you feel the next time you get burned. But it *is* possible to change the pain narrative in the future. There are psychological and sensory strategies, often called biobehavioral strategies (such as distraction, deep breathing, and engaging other senses), that can impact the chemical signals at various points in the pain pathway. If used effectively, these tactics (which we'll cover throughout this book) can lessen the level of pain you perceive. For children, being exposed to these tools early in life can be a game changer in determining how they respond to painful situations going forward. After all, children have had fewer life opportunities to learn what is and isn't painful to them, so these tactics can both lessen children's pain in the moment and prevent them from associating future potentially painful experiences with severe discomfort and anxiety.

Chronic Pain

Unlike acute pain, chronic pain is not short-lived and it does not serve as an alarm system to protect us from harm. Chronic pain is usually defined as pain lasting three months or more (though some define it as lasting at least six months) and may not be tied to any injury or tissue damage at all. For many people (both children and adults), chronic pain begins as acute pain, brought on by an injury or illness, but the pain persists even after the body recovers. In these instances, the nervous system continues to sound the pain alarm unnecessarily, like a town crier who won't stop yelling.

It's not always clear why acute pain becomes chronic, but researchers have discovered that this tends to occur when the pain pathway becomes hypersensitive, causing even small sensations to trigger pain signals to the brain. This also causes areas of the brain that sense pain and alert us to threat, like the amygdala and areas of the prefrontal cortex, to become hyperresponsive, so that the central nervous system remains flooded with emergency signals even when the source of the pain is no longer there. This concept is called central sensitization. One stark example of this is phantom limb pain, the sensation some people experience that an amputated limb is still present and aching. Though the limb and its damaged peripheral nerves are no longer part of the body, the central nervous system continues to receive pain signals.

In other cases, chronic pain may seem to develop out of nowhere, making it difficult to pinpoint when it became a consistent problem. This doesn't make it any less real. It can start with an occasional backache that announces itself with a timid twinge and then grows surreptitiously into a gnawing pang that becomes impossible to ignore. Or it can begin with intermittent yet subtle headaches that multiply in intensity and frequency after puberty hits. This is especially true for girls, who are more likely than boys to develop a chronic pain condition and who often experience its onset between the ages of twelve and fourteen, when the hormones that prompt puberty are ramping up.[7] (For a discussion of why girls—and women—are disproportionately impacted by chronic pain, see Chapter 12.)

Chronic pain can also set in as part of a disease or its treatment; with some illnesses, such as sickle cell anemia, cancer, arthritis, and Lyme disease, the pain associated with the condition can take on a life of its own. It's important to note that, in cases like this, even highly effective treatments for the underlying illness may not alleviate the pain and anxiety that go along with it. In fact, some treatments can cause further pain—think, for instance, of cancer treatments such as chemotherapy and radiation. If someone, child or adult, has a chronic illness, it's critical to treat both the underlying disease *and* the pain it brings on.

Treating that pain, however, is not as intuitive as one might think. One of the biggest misconceptions about alleviating chronic pain (of which there are many) is that it can be managed in the same way that acute pain is. Typically, acute and chronic pain require very different treatments. Unfortunately, this is something that people, even physicians, don't always realize.

But managing chronic pain *is* possible, typically through a multi-pronged approach that may or may not include medication. Researchers now understand that, while chronic pain conditions vary in their particulars, the majority of them are rooted in the same underlying neurobiological processes—and we have the ability to influence those processes. Factors such as emotions, memories, environment, sleep habits, behavior, and even our understanding of how to manage our symptoms all have important impacts on chronic pain. This means that we can use psychological and biobehavioral strategies to modify these factors and lessen the pain. Throughout this book we'll highlight the many tools that can make this possible.

Measuring Pain

Given that pain is individual, situational, and subjective, how on earth can a parent, a clinician, or even a friend understand the pain a child may be feeling? The answer is that we can't ever truly know another person's pain, and it is especially difficult to understand the pain of a baby or child who has limited power to communicate it. But measuring pain is essential when trying to help someone manage it. Fortunately, over the years, physicians and researchers have come up with useful pain-assessment tools. Though not perfect, these tools can offer a window into someone else's suffering.

One of the simplest and oldest strategies for assessing pain is the numeric pain scale. If you've ever gone to the doctor or the hospital with an injury, you may have come across this tactic. Generally, a nurse or physician will ask a standard question: How would you rate your pain on a scale from zero to ten, with zero being no pain and ten being the worst pain possible? Sometimes as they ask this, they produce a page of face diagrams that correspond to the numbers on the scale. Some pain scales are color-coded and use descriptive words along with the numbers (for example: one corresponds with "I have no pain" and ten corresponds with "Unable to move"). Regardless of the specifics, all of the scales are based on a person's "self-report," and they answer only one aspect of pain: intensity.

While a person's self-report of pain intensity is important, it doesn't fully capture the complex nature of pain or how it may shift over periods of time. And of course, clinicians can't ask infants for a self-report of their pain. Even aided by pictures, it can be difficult for young children (especially under four years old) to accurately report their pain level. It's also often impossible to ask people who are sedated, intubated, or have limited cognitive or motor function how much pain they feel. For these reasons, clinicians rely on additional strategies to assess pain beyond a person's self-report.[8]

Observing Pain Behaviors and the Body's Signals in Babies and Young Children

As simple as it may seem, observation is a critical strategy clinicians use to assess pain. The way babies and children move can tell us a lot about how they're feeling, particularly if we can also hear their nonverbal sounds, such as cries. There are specific facial expressions and body movements that reliably indicate pain, even across different species, and researchers have developed a coding system for measuring infants' pain based on these observable signals. The coded pain indicators include flailing arms, clenched fists, kicking legs, a furrowed brow, eyes that are squeezed shut, and an upper lip raised up in a grimace.[9] Parents and clinicians can also get a sense of the severity of babies' pain by noting their activity level, cries, and ability to be consoled.

Still, observing a baby's behavior, even if it's systematically coded and scored, is a subjective assessment in itself. "It's simply an observer looking at the child and trying to estimate the degree of pain," says Kanwaljeet J. S. (Sunny) Anand. Anand, a professor of pediatrics, anesthesiology, and perioperative and pain medicine at Stanford University Medical Center, has pioneered research on treating pain in infants. To get beyond this subjectivity in assessing babies' pain, researchers have begun to take into account physiological signals, such as heart rate, blood pressure, and electroencephalogram (EEG) brain monitoring, all of which are objective measures that don't rely on human observation. These techniques are most often used in neonatal intensive care units (NICUs) and in other hospital settings where patients may be unable to express their pain verbally or nonverbally.

Scientists are also studying infant cries in an effort to link specific frequencies and patterns of sound to pain and pain recovery, which they hope will enhance our understanding of what different types of infant cries mean. At this point, however, many of these pain measurement techniques have not made it out of the laboratory or specialized hospital settings. They foreshadow a future in which babies could be monitored while a machine runs a sophisticated algorithm to assess their pain levels and alerts a nurse the moment pain starts. But we are not there yet. It will likely be quite a while before we are able to take the subjectivity out of assessing pain.[10]

Asking about Characteristics of Pain

Once children can speak and express themselves, clinicians have additional ways of gaining a more complete understanding of their pain. When a child with chronic pain goes to a pain clinic, for example, a psychologist like Anna performs a thorough interview with the child and parents asking about much more than a numerical degree of pain intensity. A thorough assessment includes asking the child (and often the parents) many questions: When did you start to notice the pain? How did the pain start? How frequent is it? What patterns are there (if any) related to when it occurs? What kinds of words would you use to describe it—would you say it is burning, achy, tense, stabbing? How much does the pain interfere with normal life activities? How bothersome is the pain? The child is also usually given a picture of a body and asked to mark the places on the body where the pain is. Clinicians can use this information to help inform treatment strategies.

Part of a child's treatment may also involve keeping track of pain with a daily pain diary (in which they note when pain is felt, how much it hurts, and what type of pain it is). Although clinicians discourage kids with chronic pain from focusing too much on their discomfort, daily diaries can be very useful to patients and doctors trying to figure out which treatments are working best, which activities are triggering pain, and the influence of different factors like stress and sleep on how the child feels.[11] Studies also show that daily diaries tend to be a more reliable gauge of pain than questionnaires that ask children to think back on how they felt over the last week or month. It is often hard for kids (and adults) to remember how they felt and describe it retrospectively. Fortunately, keeping a daily diary has never been easier thanks to technology: smart phones offer convenient ways for children and teenagers to share their pain experiences with their medical providers. Some apps even offer tailored pain management suggestions.[12] While these tools are not flawless, they give children a voice, offer them a way to share how they're feeling, and validate that their pain is measurable and real.[13]

Whether you're listening to a baby's cries, observing a toddler's grimace, or talking to a teenager about the past week's headache diary, each of these tools can bring you closer to understanding a child's pain. This understanding—of both acute and chronic pain— enables you to begin managing it effectively. To learn how to do so, read on.

Chapter 2

Little Kids Won't Remember
It Anyway, Right?

*A look back at the historical lack of
pediatric pain management*

"Imagine that your baby needs major surgery," wrote Jill Lawson, of Silver Springs, Maryland, in a 1986 letter to the editor of the journal *Birth*. "You admit him to a major teaching facility with a solid reputation. Feeling foolish for even asking, you question several doctors about anesthesia. The surgical resident who brings you consent forms promises your baby will be put to sleep and you sign. Imagine finding out later that your son was cut open with *no anes thesia at all*. This is not a cut-and-slice horror movie. This is my life . . . and, as I have since discovered, it is a common practice."[1]

Shocking as it may seem, Lawson's letter about her son Jeffrey, who was born prematurely and underwent open-heart surgery in 1985 without receiving any pain medication, is not hyperbole. It is a testament to the fact that, for most of modern medical history, physicians were taught that infants could not feel pain. Due to an amalgam of misguided theories, spotty research, and cultural bias that dates back centuries, most physicians believed that infants' nervous systems were not developed enough to feel pain, and therefore it wasn't necessary to provide them with any pain management. The minority of physicians who questioned this prevailing notion were taught that, even if babies did feel pain, the potential side effects of medications such as anesthesia were too dangerous for their small systems and could result in breathing impairment, cardiac arrest, or death—a worry that persisted because anesthesia in infants was not yet well studied or regulated. Clinicians also falsely assumed that if babies felt pain in the moment, they surely wouldn't remember it later.

For those reasons, Jeffrey Lawson and many other babies who underwent surgery before the late 1980s and even into the early 1990s, were only given muscle relaxants during the procedure, which kept them from moving but left them fully conscious. This standard of care, which is dumbfounding today, was in place for decades, largely without the general public's knowledge.[2]

It was only after Jeffrey died of shock and organ failure several weeks after his 1985 surgery that his mother investigated her son's medical records and learned the full extent of the trauma he had endured—a trauma that most likely led to his death.

How could this standard of care have gone unnoticed and un-questioned for so long? There are several explanations:

· The culture surrounding modern medical professionals has long dictated that doctors know best, particularly since the late 1800s and early 1900s when medical schools began requiring extensive university education and train-ing, and professional medical societies were established. As a result, families have frequently trusted, often blindly, that physicians would do all that was medically pos-sible to treat their patients appropriately and prevent suffering.

- Pain was typically an afterthought. When a young patient's life was in danger, the priority was to keep the child alive. Comfort was not the physician's goal, especially given prevailing misconceptions about infants' ability to feel pain, and insufficient research on the safety of introducing anesthetics to their small systems. "Of all the issues I deal with, whether or not I'm hurting a child is probably the least worry because I don't do anything I don't think is necessary for their survival," said a physician quoted in a 1986 book on ethics in pediatric intensive care. Those with a greater impulse to prevent pain were often dissuaded by the specter of unknown complications from anesthetics.[3]

- Parents were discouraged from participating in their children's medical care. Even those bold enough to ask to be present during painful medical procedures were typically not allowed, and therefore remained in the dark about what transpired.[4]

- Many medical professionals were influenced by older attitudes about pain. Some doctors still viewed pain as beneficial or even necessary to spur the body's healing response—a misguided philosophy avowed late into the nineteenth century. Also, vestiges of Darwin's theory of human development, which cast children as a primitive, lower life form, lingered in the psyche of clinicians and led many to believe that children's expressions of pain were simply reflexes. This eventually paved the way for experimental infant pain research in the nineteenth and early twentieth centuries that involved pinprick and electric shock without the use of pain relief. The studies led clinicians to dismiss clear pain responses as reflexes and were used as evidence to deny infant pain perception.[5]

· Perhaps most importantly, infants and young children couldn't (and, of course, still can't) express their pain in words, nor could they verbally complain about their treatment. Though they could recoil and cry in the moment (and later research would reveal numerous physiological clues to their perceptions of pain), in a medical setting, those cries typically went unanswered.

The first-ever textbook devoted to pediatric pain was published in 1987 by husband-and-wife team Patrick J. McGrath, a pediatric psychologist, and Anita M. Unruh, an occupational therapist and social worker.[6] Both were working at Children's Hospital of Eastern Ontario in Canada when they published *Pain In Children and Adolescents,* which called for the medical community to rethink its approach to pediatric pain. It is hard to believe that no such book existed before then. The book's foreword by Ronald Melzack, a professor of psychology at McGill University, crystallizes just how desperately the book was needed. Dr. Melzack wrote:

> We like to think that the health professionals who look after children are doing everything they can to prevent pain or to relieve it as much as possible. It comes as a terrible shock, then, to find out that our ideas about pain in children are dominated by the myth that children do not feel pain as intensely as adults and therefore require fewer analgesics or none at all. In one study, more than 50% of children who underwent major surgery—including limb amputation, excision of a cancerous neck mass, and heart surgery—were not given any analgesics, and the remainder received woefully inadequate doses. These kinds of outrageous statistics are found in virtually every study that examines the treatment of severe pain in children.

Adolescents, who are the butt of another myth—that they will rapidly become drug addicts if they are given narcotic drugs for severe pain—do not fare much better.

It's been thirty-five years since Dr. Melzack wrote these words and yet, to some extent, they could be written today. A great deal has improved since then, and children in pain do typically fare better now. But it may still come as a terrible shock to many parents and clinicians that we are not in fact doing everything possible to prevent or treat children's pain. Before mapping the long way we still have to go, let's first look back to how we got here.

Children's Pain through the Centuries

To understand why it took until the 1980s for scientists and clinicians to reevaluate their approach to pain in babies and children, it's critical to explore the melting pot of belief systems that have coalesced over the centuries and infused our collective psyches with ideas about both the state of pain and the state of childhood.

For thousands of years, most ancient civilizations across the globe believed that supernatural powers had a hand in the infliction of pain. Gods and demons were thought to cause painful diseases, often in people who had sinned or were possessed by evil. Cures, therefore, were believed to come from religious figures, deities, sacrificial rites, prayers, or exorcisms. The ancient Greeks and Romans (between about 500 BCE to 250 CE) were the first in Western history to begin studying pain as a physiological state rather than a religious, spiritual, or superstitious matter. Hippocrates (about 460–370 BCE), the Greek physician widely considered the father of Western medicine, believed that pain and disease were not punishments from the gods or the work of evil spirits.[7] Instead they were caused by environmental factors in his view, and medicine should be approached as a secular discipline (a philosophy that led to what we now call science), which entailed treating both the body and the mind.[8] His teachings, therefore, helped lay the groundwork for our modern understanding of pain. But many other theories also took root along the way.

The Greek philosopher Aristotle (about 384–322 BCE) believed that pain originated in the heart, while Galen (about 130–200 CE), a Greek physician working in Rome, imagined a central nervous system and a peripheral nervous system similar to what we now know to be true. He wrote that the brain was the source of the nerves, which were connected via the spinal cord to a network of nerves that controlled the movements of muscles and limbs. This system also relayed pain messages to the brain. Seemingly ahead of his time, Galen also advised parents to ease babies' discomfort. He suggested soothing crying babies by rocking them and singing lullabies, and attending to them as needed.[9]

But opposing theories of pain—and childcare—were also influential, including the tough-it-out practices of the Spartans (1104–192 BCE) in ancient Greece, who believed that persevering through pain was a testament to one's character. One account notes that "women did not bathe the newborn children with water, as is the custom in all other countries, but with wine, to prove the temper and complexion in their bodies; from a notion they had that epileptic and weakly children waste away upon their being thus bathed, while on the contrary, those of a strong and vigorous habit acquire firmness and get a temper by it, like steel."[10] This approach, akin to the "no pain, no gain" philosophy, still endures in many cultural and medical contexts today.

Hippocrates, it should be noted, did not subscribe to the Spartan value system. He believed that infants and children were more sensitive to pain than adults and should be treated differently. For example, he encouraged treating teething pain, which was a consistent concern among parents and early healers. (The method of treatment, however—which included rubbing the baby's gums with hare's brain, chicken fat, honey, and flower oil—left something to be desired.)

Although the middle ages (from the fifth to the fifteenth century) saw a return to the belief that pain was brought on—and cured—by God or spiritual entities, the Persian polymath Avicenna (about 908–1036 CE) stood out as a modern thinker at the height of the Islamic Golden Age. He perceived that pain could be relieved through both physical and psychological strategies including herbal remedies, movement, hot baths, listening to pleasant music, and focusing on an engrossing activity. Avicenna—considered by some to be the father of modern medicine—also believed that children should be protected from pain, and that comforting babies would help their development, foreshadowing what modern-day researchers have found to be true.

The Renaissance period (between 1300 and 1600) brought a resurgence of interest in understanding the mechanics of pain and its treatment—often with an acknowledgment that babies and children were not merely little versions of adults but should be evaluated and treated differently. Still, there were many competing schools of thought on how to handle children's suffering. The first English-language book on pediatrics, *The Boke of Chyldren,* written by Thomas Phaer and published in 1544, offered many remedies for soothing babies' ailments and discomfort. Conversely, famed philosophers John Locke (1632–1704) and Jean-Jacques Rousseau

(1712–1778) wrote that children needed to be hardened in order to withstand life's adversities. Coddled children were more likely to die, they thought. One popular tactic of the time: bathing children in cold water, no matter how much they kicked and screamed through the ordeal. While this is an extreme example of conditioning, elements of this kind of authoritarian and regimented child-rearing philosophy persisted into the twentieth century.

As recently as 1928, John B. Watson, a behaviorist and former president of the American Psychology Association, warned of "the danger of too much mother love," in his popular and controversial book, *Psychological Care of Infant and Child*. He advised against responding to babies' cries or showing children affection. It's no wonder that parents today still grapple with the push-pull of the instinct to soothe versus the idea that their children should "tough it out."[11]

The Mystery of Babies' Cries

Throughout the ages (and still to the present day), philosophers, doctors, and parents have struggled with yet another puzzle: how to decipher babies' cries and understand what they're feeling. Crying is one of an infant's primary means of communication. Indeed, the word infant comes from the Latin *infans,* which means "one who cannot speak" or "speechless." Without the words to explain the meaning behind their cries, infants have had to rely on adults to interpret—and those interpretations have run the gamut.

In 1838, Samuel Smiles, a Scottish author and social reformer who also practiced medicine, published his book *Physical Education; Or, The Nurture and Management of Children, Founded On The Study Of Their Nature and Constitution*. His view was that babies' cries weren't typically cause for concern and were actually often beneficial for their health. "Sickly and weak children cry a great deal, and but for this, it is almost certain they would not live long," he argued. "It is their only exercise, often in fact their only nourishment, for when they cease to cry they soon sink and expire."[12]

Others, however, recognized that infants' cries, and also their facial expressions, could indicate pain—as modern scientists including Heidelise Als and Ruth Grunau have since elucidated (as discussed in Chapter 4). The pediatrician Louis Starr, the first professor of pediatrics at the University of Pennsylvania Medical School, believed it was in fact crucial to address a baby's cries because they were typically a sign of pain, distress, or illness. "The vocal sound, termed crying, is the chief if not the only means that the young infant possesses of indicating his displeasure, discomfort or suffering," he wrote in *Diseases of the Digestive Organs in Infancy and Childhood*, originally published in 1886. "Even long after the powers of speech have been developed, the cry continues to be the main channel of complaint. It may be accepted, as a rule, that a healthy child never cries. Of course, some acute pain, as from a fall or accident or blow, will cause crying in the most healthy child, but the storm is quickly over. Nothing like frequent, peevish crying or fretfulness is compatible with health."[13]

Fortunately, viewpoints like Dr. Starr's have prevailed. In the mid- and late 1900s, renowned pediatricians and child development experts Benjamin Spock and T. Berry Brazelton began revolutionizing our understanding of what babies could feel and communicate. In their bestselling books (including Dr. Spock's *Baby and Child Care*, 1946, and Dr. Brazelton's *Babies and Mothers*, 1969, and *To Listen to a Child*, 1984) both urged readers to be attentive to children's cries and other cues, to recognize their psychological and physical needs, and to respond with compassion. While their primary focus was not on pediatric pain, Dr. Spock and Dr. Brazelton popularized the notion of babies as complex individuals and advocated for their interests in medical settings and in the home.[14]

The Invention of Anesthesia and the Advent of a New Age in Pain Control

A tectonic shift in attitudes about pain came in the mid-1800s with the invention of inhaled anesthesia, which used ether nitrous oxide or chloroform to sedate patients during surgery, and later, mothers during childbirth. Up until that point, surgeons had been conditioned to tolerate their patients' shrieks and flails throughout what many described as a butchering process. But the invention of anesthesia freed patients and physicians from the sheer torture of surgery and radically transformed expectations about what medicine could offer. Now there was a salve for suffering. In 1846, at Massachusetts General Hospital, the first surgery was successfully completed using ether anesthesia. Henry Jacob Bigelow, a Harvard professor of surgery, was there to observe it and afterward pronounced: "Our craft has, once for all, been robbed of its terrors!"[15]

The invention of anesthesia was a seminal event, propelling the study of pain management forward and elevating its medical value. But it would be decades before physicians and scientists developed a more complete understanding of pain in its myriad forms, and indeed that endeavor is still unfinished. We now know that pain is a phenomenon that is at once physiological, psychological, scientific, subjective, and emotional, but many mysteries remain. What's more, it has taken years to learn how to decipher and respond appropriately to the nonverbal cues of babies and young children—and clinicians and researchers are still learning. It has taken longer still for the modern medical establishment to prioritize the study and treatment of pain in our youngest patients. For that last step, we have Jill Lawson and several trailblazing researchers to thank.

Jeffrey Lawson's Legacy

Jeffrey Lawson's life was cut tragically short in 1985, after he underwent open-heart surgery without receiving any anesthesia, but his legacy lives on. His mother, Jill Lawson, spoke out publicly about her son's trauma and, in so doing, she pulled back the curtain on the often barbaric medical protocols that were commonplace in the operating room.

In her 1986 letter in *Birth,* Lawson described the horror: "Jeffrey had holes cut on both sides of his neck, another hole cut in his right chest, an incision from his breastbone around to his backbone, his ribs pried apart, and an extra artery near his heart tied off. This was topped off with another hole cut in his left side for a chest tube. The operation lasted 1 ½ hours. Jeffrey was awake through it all."

After he died, when Lawson asked the anesthesiologist why she had given Jeffrey a paralytic during surgery but had not given him pain medicine, the doctor "said Jeffrey was too sick to tolerate powerful anesthetics," wrote Lawson. "Anyway, she said, it had never been demonstrated to her that premature babies feel pain. She seemed sincerely puzzled as to why I was concerned."

Lawson was not just concerned, she was outraged, and she made it her mission to change the status quo of pediatric pain management by writing to every relevant medical society and journal she could find. After the Lawsons' story got picked up by major news outlets, it sparked public outcry and inspired researchers to focus on pediatric pain.

Lawson's advocacy, along with the groundbreaking work of a handful of scientists and physicians practicing in those years, is rightfully credited with helping to launch a movement that would yield major advancements in the field of pediatric pain in a very short time. As compared to the beginning of the 1980s, the number of papers published annually on children's pain management had doubled by the end of the decade, and a sea change was underway in how clinicians treated children and addressed their pain.[16]

"The modern field of pediatric pain was born out of a marriage of science and public concern," recalls Dr. McGrath, who is now an emeritus professor of psychiatry at Dalhousie University, and vice president of research, innovation, and knowledge translation for the IWK Health Centre in Halifax, Canada. One indicator of how swiftly the tide turned as a result of that marriage of medicine and activism was the title of a 1986 *Washington Post* article inspired by the Lawsons' experience: "Surgery Without Anesthesia: Can Preemies Feel Pain?" Presenting both sides of that debate, and evaluating whether newborns could withstand the potentially negative effects of anesthesia, the piece included quotes from doctors skeptical about changing their practices. One anesthesiologist, considering the risk of administering a depressant to a "very small preemie," had this to say: "I don't know if I have a body of knowledge that tells me if they don't perceive or feel pain or if there are differences from older children and adults. . . . But I'm not going to be knocking off babies because someone says I'm torturing them."[17]

Just one year later, however, after Jill Lawson had awakened the world to the living nightmare many babies suffered during surgery, both the American Academy of Pediatrics and the American Society of Anesthesiologists put forth their first statements acknowledging the need for adequate anesthetic agents for newborns during surgery.[18] Of course, these 1987 recommendations did not instantly change the practices of all physicians, nor did they immediately transform the culture surrounding the medical care of babies and children. Still, they marked the dawning of a new era.[19]

The Birth of the Scientific Study of Pediatric Pain

One of the researchers at the forefront of this revolutionary era was Kanwaljeet J. S. (Sunny) Anand, who recalls he came to the field in 1983 "quite by accident when doing research as a Rhodes Scholar at the University of Oxford." Today, Dr. Anand is a professor of pediatrics, anesthesiology, and perioperative and pain medicine at Stanford University Medical Center. Back then, he was tasked with studying how anesthesia given to mothers during birth affected their newborns, and quickly discovered that there was very little research on the effects of anesthesia given directly to newborns themselves.

"At the same time, I'd been working in the newborn ICU, and I would see my patients come back from surgery with severe clinical instability," says Dr. Anand. "It seemed the babies were doing fairly well before the surgery, and they would come back with a big change in their physiology, which was really distressing but also puzzling to me. So I started thinking maybe that was the effects of the anesthesia given or the effects of the surgery, and that's when I realized that there was no anesthesia being given. Babies were having surgery without anesthetic because it was commonly believed and commonly taught everywhere that babies don't feel pain."

Though Dr. Anand could see that babies reacted to painful stimuli in the neonatal intensive care unit (the insertion of an IV line, for instance), he had been taught that their reactions were likely the result of a reflex rather than a perception of pain. "A lot of text-books said that, because babies' nerves are not myelinated, their pain system may not be capable of transmitting the stimulus to the brain," he says. "Of course, when I talked to experienced mothers it was very clear that they knew babies felt pain. But there was no objective proof."

Through a series of studies, Dr. Anand produced the proof. First, with his Oxford advisor Sir Albert Ansley-Green, he designed an observational pilot study in which he analyzed blood samples taken from babies before and after surgery. "Our hypothesis was that because babies are immature, they would have a much lower hormonal response to surgery as compared to older children or adults," he says. The results, which were published in the journal *Hormone Research* in 1985 (the same year as Jeffrey Lawson's surgery), surprised Dr. Anand. "The babies' stress response was five times that of adults undergoing a similar surgery. I thought, maybe they're feeling pain, and that's why they have these huge stress responses."[20]

The results were so remarkable that Dr. Ansley-Green readily agreed to a change in Dr. Anand's research focus, shifting it to studying babies' stress response to surgery. Next, the two scientists designed randomized trials that compared the blood samples of babies who received adequate anesthesia during surgery (the experimental group) to samples from babies subject to the standard surgical care at the time (the control group), who received considerably less anesthesia. Dr. Anand is quick to point out that even the control group of babies in his study received some pain medicine during surgery. "The fact that babies at the time were not getting anesthetic during surgery was just not acceptable to me. I just couldn't come to terms with it," he says.

The results of those trials were first published in the medical journal *The Lancet* in January 1987.[21] As Dr. Anand summarizes them, "the babies who were given proper anesthetic prior to surgery had stress responses that were markedly lower, those babies were a lot more stable after the surgery, and had fewer complications." This finding was pivotal and lent credence to Lawson's crusade to ensure that babies undergoing surgery would receive adequate anesthesia.

Dr. Anand followed up this research with another analysis on the perception of pain in infants, which he published in the *New England Journal of Medicine* with Paul Hickey, now chief of anesthesiology at Boston Children's Hospital and professor of anesthesia at Harvard Medical School. The research, conducted while Dr. Anand was doing his postdoctoral work at Harvard Medical School, was a review of all the infant literature related to pain, and it showed, at long last, that infants are not only capable of mounting a physiological response to painful stimuli, they are capable of perceiving pain—*and* their behaviors indicate that they can remember it.[22]

"But I still felt that people would not be convinced that giving anesthetic to babies is a good thing unless we show that it changes mortality rates after surgery and improves survival," says Dr. Anand. Physicians were justifiably concerned that anesthesia could be harmful to babies, says Dr. Anand, but he believed that some of the concern was outdated and based on older incarnations of anesthetics that offered less controlled dosing. So Dr. Anand set out to prove that giving anesthesia to babies both reduced their pain and reduced their risk of death.

He and Dr. Hickey designed a randomized, placebo-controlled, double-blind trial (the most rigorous type of study) comparing an experimental group of infants who received a high-dose opiate anesthetic during heart surgery and a continuous infusion of analgesia post-operatively to a control group of infants who received a much lower dose of anesthetic, designed to approximate what was then the standard of care. The results were definitive: "In our control group we had a mortality rate of 27 percent, which was typical at the time. In our experimental group, there was a *zero* percent mortality. That sent a shockwave through the anesthesia pediatric community," says Dr. Anand. "It was proof that giving anesthetic reduced mortality and other complications."[23]

A Calling to Make Kids' Lives Better

As Dr. Anand was conducting his studies in the 1980s, several other researchers began immersing themselves in this new field of pediatric pain medicine and founding pain centers devoted exclusively to children. On the West Coast, in 1985, Donald C. Tyler and Elliot Krane, who were both at the University of Washington and Seattle Children's Hospital at the time, founded a pediatric pain management program. On the East Coast, in 1986, Charles Berde founded the Pain Treatment Center for acute and chronic pain management for children at Boston Children's Hospital, and Neil Schechter founded the pediatric pain clinic for acute and chronic pain management at Connecticut Children's Medical Center in Hartford.

Around the same time, innovators in the field of pediatric nursing were also studying pain in children and how to best measure and manage it in hospitals and other medical settings. Joann "Jo" Eland, a nurse and psychologist, began contributing to the literature as early as the 1970s with her published master's thesis about the paucity of pediatric pain management, and soon produced more on how children communicate pain.[24] She ultimately dedicated her career at the University of Iowa to that research and to educating nurses about pain in children—even advocating for children's pain management around the world. Other nurse leaders, such as Judith Beyer at the University of Missouri-Kansas City School of Nursing, continued this mission in the 1980s and 1990s by establishing practice guidelines and standards for measuring pain in children with painful conditions such as sickle cell disease.[25] She also focused on tailoring tools for children of different racial and ethnic backgrounds. These early research and clinical efforts by nurses to provide comfort and care to suffering children were invaluable to the emerging field of pediatric pain.

In those early days, some clinicians were motivated by the chance to explore uncharted scientific territory, while others were drawn to the field because they saw a critical need for it, and some practitioners were driven by both factors. Anesthesiologist Allen Finley says the inspiration to devote his life to pediatric pain management was a four-year-old girl named Caitlyn.

Dr. Finley, who is now a professor of anesthesia, pain management, and perioperative medicine at Dalhousie University and medical director of pediatric pain management at IWK Health Centre, met Caitlyn in 1989 in the hospital where she was dying of cancer. When he began treating her, "she was curled up under the blankets in agony, like a wet dishrag," he says. "She was not talking, reacting, or interacting with her family or the world."

Dr. Finley knew that Caitlyn had only a little time left to live and that she was in excruciating pain, so he decided to try something fairly radical: "I managed her with a continuous intravenous infusion of morphine, which nobody had ever thought about doing before in a child, at least in our center. And that kept her happy, playing, singing, and telling jokes until the night she died," says Dr. Finley.

How could it be a radical idea to alleviate the suffering of a terminally ill child? "There was no culture of treating pain as an entity for adults or children then, but particularly not for children," explains Dr. Finley. "Pain management basically didn't go out of the operating room at that time." A 1986 study led by Neil Schechter, now director of the chronic pain clinic at Boston Children's Hospital and associate professor of anesthesia at Harvard Medical School, found that children in hospitals received half the pain medicine doses administered to adults with the same diagnosis. Among the children, infants and younger kids were less likely to be given any pain medication than older ones.[26] Other work led by Dr. Schechter explored physicians' attitudes toward pain in children, and found some of their beliefs contributing to the undertreatment of pediatric pain.[27]

Caitlyn showed Dr. Finley the transformative power of appropriate pain management for children. After receiving morphine, Caitlyn was able to be the little girl she'd been before devastating illness had taken over her body. "That gave her family six weeks more with the child they knew before she died, and it got her home for Christmas and New Year's," says Dr. Finley, who still displays on his wall a picture Caitlyn made of a rainbow one day at the hospital. "She changed my life completely."

Dr. Finley says that his experience treating Caitlyn is what led him to work with Patrick McGrath, who had coauthored the first textbook on pediatric pain, published just two years prior. "There was no formal training in pain education so it wasn't until Caitlyn that I really saw this as something I had to do," says Dr. Finley, who spent the next years working with Dr. McGrath at Dalhousie University and IWK Health Centre hospital to overhaul how children's pain was managed across disciplines and medical specialties.[28] While Dr. Finley began by addressing pain in pediatric palliative care (end of life cases, like Caitlyn's), he went on to establish the practice of giving children adequate anesthesia for hospital procedures, such as bone marrow biopsies. "It grew into acute pain and chronic pain across other services in the hospital, and then we realized that we needed a proper service with a multidisciplinary team," says Finley. In 1995 he cofounded, with Dr. McGrath, the Centre for Pediatric Pain Research in Halifax.

The centers in Halifax, Boston, Hartford, and Seattle became breeding grounds for pediatric pain research, and the influence of their work spread as these early researchers mentored junior scientists—who in turn developed their own expertise in pediatric pain and mentored the next generation of pediatric pain researchers and clinicians. These incubators of scientific progress would eventually birth important developments in the study of pediatric pain.

A Growing Research Movement

In 1988, Drs. Taylor and Krane hosted the first meeting of what would become the International Symposium of Pediatric Pain in Seattle, Washington. Two years later, the Special Interest Group (SIG) on Pain in Childhood was established as part of the International Association for the Study of Pain. While the Pain in Childhood SIG was a small group at first, not many more than a dozen members, those involved in the early years shaped the future of the field. They included Canadians Carl von Baeyer, Allen Finley, Ruth Grunau, and Celeste Johnston; Americans Charles Berde, Elliot Krane, Neil Schechter, Gary Walco, and Lonnie Zeltzer; and international members such as Gunnar L. Olsson, Maria Fitzgerald, Eeva-Liisa Maunuksela, Linda Franck, and Ricardo Carbajal, among others. The Pain in Childhood SIG now stands as the academic and intellectual home to hundreds of scientists working in this field.

In addition to conducting first-of-its kind research and advocating for children, pediatric pain scientists and clinicians saw the importance of providing training to medical providers and researchers in other fields who were interested in learning more about pediatric pain. A group of dedicated Canadians led the effort to formalize interdisciplinary training and established the Pain in Child Health (PICH) international research training initiative.[29] Since 2002, this program has brought together international trainees from nursing, psychology, medicine, and the basic sciences to learn about the obstacles confronting pediatric pain research and delve into approaches for studying pediatric pain processes and solutions. Over the course of the past two decades, this educational program has linked trainees from around the world with senior research leaders in the field. It has made it possible for say, a graduate student from the University of Georgia to connect with Dr. Kenneth Craig, of the University of British Columbia, who is an innovator in the study of nonverbal assessment of pain and the social aspects of pain in children. Similarly, a trainee from the University of Bath in the UK might have the opportunity to get to know the cutting-edge treatment research being conducted by Dr. Tonya Palermo in her Seattle lab. Importantly, this program has inspired researchers (Anna included) to continue working in the field. Recent data analysis shows that PICH trainees have contributed significantly to the scientific literature on pediatric pain, which improves our understanding of children's acute and chronic pain and our ability to treat it.

With the groundwork established, the field of pediatric pain has been able to become increasingly specialized, with researchers now actively addressing a range of specific issues with direct impact on care for children. Among them:

- How to effectively share knowledge with hospitals and in community settings about the importance of treating acute pain in children and reducing pain associated with vaccinations and minor medical procedures.
- Why some children develop chronic pain after an acute musculoskeletal injury or illness while others do not.
- What role sleep plays in the development of chronic pain in children.
- How children's memories about past pain shape their subsequent experiences involving pain, and how we can use these processes to reduce pain and related anxiety.
- How best to treat chronic pain in children using both medical and psychological interventions, and how to help their parents support them.
- How pain affects families across generations (Anna's primary area of focus).
- What innovative ways can be found to measure pain in babies and children of all ages.
- What refinements can be made in the use of pain medications after children undergo surgery.
- How parents influence a child's perception of pain, and how to effectively harness their impact.
- How pain management can be improved for children with cancer and other chronic illnesses.

Over the last three decades, this small yet growing group of dedicated scientists and clinicians has put pediatric pain management on the map, and there are now at least forty multidisciplinary pediatric pain clinics in North America. Even so, their important contributions—and the field in general—are still flying woefully under the radar. The primary reasons for this? It typically takes years for research findings to move beyond the lab and into clinical practice.[30] What's more, cultural norms and medical dogma are not easily refashioned. Centuries of misconceptions about both children and pain are enshrined in hard-to-break habits. To this day, physicians and medical students receive only a handful of education hours devoted to pain management, in adults or children, throughout their general training.[31] This has led to significant gaps in what most physicians know about how to treat pain effectively. And as we've learned, when patients are unable to verbalize their pain, it is often ignored.

This inertia has meant that the crusade for better pain management for children worldwide continues. Many efforts are making headway. Consider the work of ChildKind International, organized between 2008 and 2010 by Dr. Schechter at Harvard and several colleagues, including Dr. Finley at Dalhousie. ChildKind International is an organization that recognizes and certifies hospitals that have made an institutional commitment—philosophically and practically—to providing evidence-based pediatric pain prevention, assessment, and relief. "What we needed was a cultural shift and it starts with the notion that generous, thoughtful, and kind people make a difference from the bottom up," Dr. Schechter says. "The program and the certification process are about creating institutional change through policies, procedures, and protocols that promote a child's comfort, and transform the culture surrounding pediatric pain management at that hospital."

Dr. Christine Chambers, at Dalhousie University, recently launched the Solutions for Kids in Pain (SKIP) program, dedicated to disseminating research findings about managing pain in children to those who need them most: hospitals, pediatric medical providers, and parents. The mission of the program is to drive more implementation in practice of evidence-based solutions and give more children access to treatments researchers have found to be effective. SKIP currently operates only in Canada, but serves as a model that could be replicated in other countries.[32]

Dr. Finley, who has spent decades lecturing globally to help establish pediatric pain best practices, has indeed seen a cultural shift. "In the early days, people thought that pain treatment in children might be too dangerous, or children wouldn't feel pain or remember it, so they didn't want to take the chance. Even twenty years ago, when I'd go to other countries, practitioners would say, 'What? You mean children really have pain?' But we've overcome a lot of that," he says. "Then, fifteen years ago, I'd lecture in different countries and hospital staff would say, 'Oh, yeah, we think children probably have pain, but we don't know what to do about it.' And then ten years ago it was, 'Yeah, we know what to do about pediatric pain, and we're trying to get it implemented, but we're not sure how.' So there are all these steps along the way and it happens at different rates in different places and with different people."

The Next Frontier In Pediatric Pain Management

At major hospitals in North America today, there is no doubt that pain protocols surrounding pediatric surgeries have vastly improved since Jeffrey Lawson's case made headlines in 1986. Further, it's partly because of the pain management practices now in place that surgical outcomes in children have improved, as well. As an example, we can look to the case of Talia, who suffered near-fatal heart failure days after her birth in 2008 in a New York City hospital. Diagnosed with a heart defect, she underwent open-heart surgery but was given adequate anesthesia. Her pain was also managed throughout her post-operative care, and during subsequent surgeries and medical procedures as she got older. Her parents were allowed to be with her regularly while she was in the hospital—no doubt easing her response to pain both emotionally and physiologically, as research has established that a parent's presence typically does.

Just as Jill Lawson had believed her baby would be sedated appropriately, Talia's mother, Rachel Goldberg, assumed that pain medicine would be given as needed. But unlike Lawson, Goldberg's assumption was accurate. The Goldbergs (and countless other patients) have benefited from the lessons of the past, and at this writing, Talia is thirteen years old and thriving.

"But we're not where we need to be with pain management," cautions Dr. Finley, referring to both adults and children. Not only is there a need for more physician education regarding pain management, there is also a need for parent education and awareness. In the same way that medical errors are not tolerated, untreated pain also should not be tolerated. "It's an incident report and an investigation if somebody falls out of a hospital bed because the bed rail wasn't up, or if somebody gets a central line infection or an overdose of a medication. Well, it should also be an investigation if somebody gets an underdose of pain medication," says Dr. Finley. "The failure to treat pain in a hospital should be an adverse event, and when it happens, the system should look for ways to improve."

We should also continue to look for every opportunity to improve the management of chronic pain in children, which, even today, some physicians don't recognize affects kids. A child with chronic pain will typically visit a series of medical professionals— usually over the course of one to two years—before finding appropriate treatment through a specialist or a team of clinicians at a pediatric pain center.[33] Some children never find that treatment at all.

We are lucky that we live in a time that has seen so much improvement, but we must not lose sight of how far we have yet to go. Scientists and clinicians now know enough to reduce the burden of pain dramatically in children of all ages. But it's up to both medical practitioners and parents to push for better. And it's possible. As we saw with Jeffrey Lawson, when parents, medical professionals, and the media join together, we have enormous power to make change.

Chapter 3

Ouch!

Easing the sting of shots

Many parents feel anxious about their babies' first shots. Nobody wants to see their child in pain, and Rachel was no different. After giving birth to her first child, Lena, Rachel had barely figured out how to pack her diaper bag and unfold her stroller before she was faced with the task of getting her newborn to the pediatrician's office and soothing her through her vaccinations. But Rachel was fortunate that, as a health journalist, she had already learned a lot about what she could do to help her baby. She'd read studies led by Anna Taddio, a professor of pharmacy at the University of Toronto, who has spent much of her career researching how to reduce childhood pain during vaccinations and other medical procedures. Rachel had also spoken with Dr. Taddio, who'd emphasized that there are lots of easy things parents can do to lessen the trauma of shots for their children.

Dr. Taddio and her colleagues have conducted a number of studies revealing that commonsense strategies—such as holding your baby on your lap (as opposed to having her lie on her back on the examination table) and allowing her to nurse or be fed by bottle, or suck on a pacifier or cloth soaked in sugar-water solution—can substantially reduce pain response during vaccinations.[1] "The combination of the physical comfort, the sweet taste, and the sucking—which is a baby's primal instinct—takes the baby's attention away from the injection and results in less crying," says Dr. Taddio. It certainly worked for Rachel and her baby. During all of Lena's shots she was so busy being hugged and fed that she never made a peep. When Rachel compared her vaccination experiences to the screams she heard from infants getting their shots in nearby exam rooms, she couldn't understand why more people didn't use the simple—seemingly magical—strategies she'd learned.

She soon found out that these scientifically proven tactics had not (and still have not) made their way into many clinicians' offices. Fewer than 5 percent of children receive any type of pain intervention during vaccinations. Large numbers of parents aren't aware that any strategies exist and therefore don't know to ask about them. Even when parents *do* express a desire to see pain relieved during shots, they are often met with resistance.

Rachel eventually experienced pushback herself when she tried to ease the pain of vaccinations for her younger daughter, Annika, during her first shots as an infant. Having moved to a new town, Rachel discovered that her new pediatrician had not gotten the memo about Dr. Taddio's work. At her first appointment, the nurse stopped Rachel from allowing Annika to sit on her lap and suck on sugar-water or a bottle, during her shots, saying she feared Annika would choke (a nearly impossible outcome under the circumstances). Rachel explained that she'd used these established pain-relief methods with her older child at her previous pediatrician's office and they had worked beautifully. But the nurse insisted on administering the vaccinations without any pain relief, and as a result, Annika became one of the screaming babies Rachel remembered hearing in other exam rooms. At their second vaccination appointment, Rachel came armed with printouts of Dr. Taddio's studies to show the medical staff. Surely, she thought, they'd let her use these interventions with the proof of their efficacy in hand. Once again, the nurse resisted, but she ultimately acquiesced. Later that day, however, the pediatrician called to reprimand Rachel for undermining the nurses. The pediatrician clearly did not understand the vulnerable position in which he was putting his young patients and their parents—nor did he recognize the importance of minimizing childhood pain.

Rachel wasted no time in switching pediatricians. But there are countless other pediatricians with similar attitudes in towns across the country. Some might ask, what's the big deal? It's just a few needle pricks, right? Wrong. Early pain exposures have great import. "The impact of repeated pain during injections can lead people to have fears of doctors and needles for the rest of their lives," says Dr. Taddio.[2]

The Aftershocks of Poorly Managed Needle Pricks

In the United States, about three hundred million doses of vaccinations are given in a typical year (exclusive of Covid-19 vaccinations), the vast majority of them to children. Children receive about fifty-four doses of various vaccines by the time they are eighteen, although some of these are combined to require fewer separate shots than this.[3] While there is no doubt that vaccines save lives, keeping us safe from deadly and debilitating diseases through individual and herd immunity, in many cases the injections are children's first painful experiences. These pokes and our responses to them have the power to influence children's nerve signaling. And when vaccination pain is improperly managed, it can have detrimental effects on how children react to subsequent pain—and how they feel about medical care—as they grow up.

Dr. Taddio's research has found that more than 60 percent of children and nearly 25 percent of adults report a fear of needles. For eight percent of children and seven percent of adults, that fear is the main reason they don't get vaccinations, even though this creates dangers for their health and the health of their communities. For some people, needle fear can develop into a needle phobia (an extreme fear of needles), which tends to persist unless it is treated.[4]

It follows, then, that proactive pain control during vaccinations can do more than just ease crying in the moment; it can go a long way toward preventing heightened responses to pain and medical phobias that may cause people to resist getting the medical care they need. In other words, if more medical practices acknowledged the need to manage pain during routine childhood immunizations, and actively addressed parents' concerns and anxieties for their children (often stemming from their own pasts), it could very well alleviate many people's aversions to receiving necessary vaccinations and procedures.

The notion that needle prick pain should be managed in babies and children is so new even to medical professionals that as recently as 2016, the American Academy of Pediatrics (AAP) released an updated policy statement emphasizing the need for improved and consistent pain control for newborns during minor medical procedures. The AAP committee members noted that repeated exposure to pain early in life (from procedures such as vaccinations and heel sticks, for instance) can create short- *and* long-term changes in brain development and in the body's stress response systems. After decades of research, the AAP has come to the firm conclusion that needle pain in young children matters, and recommends that caregivers and healthcare providers take steps to prevent and reduce this pain.[5]

Reducing Acute Pain

The pain you feel from a needle injection is classified as acute pain. In this scenario, as the needle breaks through the skin, it activates nerve endings called nociceptors, which rapidly fire pain messages through the spinal cord—via the ascending pain pathway—to the brain. Along the way, the pain messages pass through a number of areas of the brain that control autonomic functions, such as heart rate and breathing, so the experience of pain is often accompanied by feelings of distress, anxiety, and fear—a process that has evolved to alert us that we need to move or get away from painful stimuli.

But we are not powerless against this cascade of pain messages. We can employ a range of strategies to influence how the brain interprets the pain signals it receives. (For instance, based on the inputs and messages the brain receives, it might decide: "Danger! Danger! You're being attacked by a giant needle!" Or, it may decide: "Oh, there's that little silver poking stick again. It will sting for a few seconds and then it will go away.") If the pain-relieving strategies are carried out effectively, the brain can dampen the chemical messages it sends back down through the descending pain pathway, which can quell the pain response and related distress.

In short: injections don't have to trigger severe pain or anxiety, and if we start using these pain-relieving tactics early in life, they will become integrated into children's responses to pain as their brains mature.

Proven Pain-Relief Strategies for Injections

· Position the baby or child in a caregiver's arms or on a parent's lap.

· Let the baby or child suck on a sweet solution (a cloth or pacifier dipped in sugar water).

· Breastfeed or bottle-feed before or during the injection.

· Encourage the child (if old enough) to practice relaxation and deep-breathing exercises.

· Use distraction techniques.

· Apply a numbing cream to the child's skin before the procedure.

Hold your child

One of the best things about the pain relief approaches outlined here is that they are not complicated to understand, learn, or implement. Most of them have been used intuitively for a long time. Certainly this is true of holding babies to comfort them during episodes of pain and stress, which mothers have done since the beginning of time. Research in the past two decades provides the scientific explanation of how cuddling calms the nerves, particularly when babies are cuddled skin-to-skin with their caregiver. This physical contact helps regulate infant heart rate, lowers stress hormone levels, and helps reduce crying and distress.[6]

Let your child suck on a sweet solution or breastfeed

Another age-old pain-reduction technique is that of giving babies a sweet solution during procedures. For example, it is tradition for a mohel, who is trained to perform Jewish ritual circumcisions, to give a baby boy a few drops of sweet wine (or a small cloth dipped in sugar water) to taste while performing the procedure. Similarly, nurses have been sneaking sugar solutions to babies in hospitals for years. But it wasn't until the late 1980s and 1990s that researchers began testing this method of pain reduction in earnest. In controlled studies, they compared responses to needle pain when babies had sugar water during injections and when they didn't. These studies reveal that, overwhelmingly, babies exhibit less perception of pain when they are given a sugary solution during injections. Breast-feeding and skin-to-skin contact during vaccinations have similar effects—and have the bonus effect of triggering the release of oxy-tocin (a feel-good hormone that can reduce distress and increase pain tolerance). The same exact injection can be made into a less painful experience for a baby simply by providing access to the mother's breast—or, if that is not possible, to a bottle or cloth dipped in sugar water.[7]

Engage your child in relaxation exercises

The American Academy of Pediatrics recommends several behavioral strategies to ease pain during routine medical procedures. These techniques include relaxation and breathing exercises and guided imagery activities (such as helping a child imagine a calming scene), which can slow heart rates and help children focus their attention on their breath or on an imaginary world instead of the pain. For young children, parents might even bring in bubbles to blow, which will facilitate deep breathing.[8]

Distract your child in other pleasant ways

Simple distraction—with a song, book, or video game—can also ease anxiety and discomfort during an injection. In 2014, a review by researchers at Dalhousie University of all studies performed up to that date relating to distraction during vaccinations, concluded that it was effective at reducing pain and distress. This meta-analysis also highlighted that children are more likely to report less pain and upset when the distraction is more interactive than passive (for example, when they are engaging with a smart device or playing a game rather than watching a video). Whatever the task, if it draws the brain's focus to something other than the shot, the body's pain modulation system suppresses the pain response and the interpretation of the nerve signals is not as painful. Distraction therefore doesn't only help children ignore pain signaling—it actually *changes* pain signaling.[9]

Apply a topical anesthetic in advance

While topical anesthetics are rarely used for this purpose in American doctor's offices, it is common in Canada and Europe to apply a cream or patch (typically lidocaine) to numb the area of an injection in advance. The effect is to prevent the nociceptive nerves from firing in the first place. Note, however, that this approach does nothing to engage the descending pain-control pathway that inhibits pain signaling and distress. Even with a numb arm, an older child can still see the needle coming, remember prior experiences, and experience anxiety.[10]

Which of these pain relief strategies is most effective? Lindsey Cohen, professor of psychology at Georgia State University and director of the Children's Health and Medical Pain (CHAMP) lab in Atlanta, has been studying that question. His research is focused on identifying the best methods for reducing immunization pain for children of different ages. One of the first studies Dr. Cohen conducted in this area followed a group of fourth graders who received three immunization injections at their school health clinic over a six-month period in 1999. The children were randomly assigned to three groups, distinguished by the type of treatment they would receive across all three shots: each time, the first group was distracted with a movie (with the school nurse not only instructing them to watch it but also asking questions about what was happening in it); the second group had a topical numbing cream applied an hour in advance (the necessary time for it to take full effect); and the third group received "typical care" by the school nurse (with no special pain-relief strategy employed). As injections were administered, all by the same nurse, the children's responses were videotaped and coded to measure their distress and coping levels. The study found that the kids who were distracted by the movie exhibited less distress and more coping behaviors (such as deep breathing) than those in the other two groups. Children who were given the numbing cream showed the most distress, perhaps because their anticipation levels had risen during the hour between its application and the shot.[11]

Dr. Cohen's research lab found a similar pattern in a study with infants (7.5 months old on average) receiving a routine immunization. Here, too, the babies were randomly assigned to receive distraction, topical numbing cream, or typical care—and again the finding was that the lowest level of distress, on average, was exhibited by those who were distracted.[12]

Memory Matters

Still not convinced that these interventions can have real impact on children? Consider that we are all biologically programmed to avoid injuries to ourselves, and one of the ways we do this is by remembering and learning from painful experiences. The child getting a shot is no exception; it hurts, and the brain carefully saves that information for later reference. Moreover, to the extent that an experience is emotionally charged, the memory of it tends to be stronger.

So, when a child experiences a high level of distress as part of getting a shot, that injection—and the pain that went along with it—is more likely to be remembered, and that memory will inform the child's feelings about subsequent medical procedures.

Interestingly, the memories themselves may matter most in this context—and memories can get distorted. Research led by Melanie Noel, an associate professor of clinical psychology at the University of Calgary, in Alberta, Canada, has shown that children's memories of pain intensity often differ from how they initially rated that pain—and their subsequent pain response to an equivalent event is closer to the memory than the initial rating. For example, in one of her studies, published in the journal *Pain,* children aged eight to twelve years old were exposed to a painful stimulus—in this case, submerging their hand in ice-cold water (called the cold pressor task)—and rated the pain level they experienced. Two weeks later, the kids were asked to rate that painful task based only on their memories. Some children remembered the pain as more severe than it felt at the time while others remembered it as less severe. Another two weeks later, the children repeated the same pain task and again rated its intensity. It turned out that those who had remembered the pain to be more intense than they had rated it the first time now assigned a higher pain intensity to the second experience. The implication in general is that a child who remembers a past shot as worse than it was is likely to respond to subsequent shots more negatively than a child who remembers a past shot as a minor event. "We know that pain isn't over when the needle ends," says Dr. Noel. "How children remember painful experiences can follow them throughout life."[13]

Fortunately, memories can be influenced. In one study published in the *Journal of Pediatric Psychology,* children were able to forget aspects of a painful experience by remembering positive details about that event, such as receiving a favorite cartoon sticker. As a result, they were less anxious about an upcoming painful event and better able to cope with it. This research indicates that parents can affect a child's future pain response by reshaping their memories of the past. For example, a parent might prompt a child to recall the sweet lollipop she had during a vaccination, or the song they sang together, thereby shifting the focus of that memory and aiding in forgetting the pain.[14]

"Kids' memories are so malleable and plastic, we've found that simply talking with kids about their needle experiences afterward can actually change their memory of it," says Dr. Noel. "So after an injection, you want to highlight the things you'd like the child to remember, and build their confidence in their ability to handle these experiences. You could tell a child, 'You were so brave! You did so well taking deep breaths, and that really helped!' Or 'Remember looking at the video on my phone? That's called distraction and you actually know how to do it!' These narratives help reframe the memory in a positive light and build children's self-efficacy for the next time."

Dr. Noel likes to think of this memory reframing as a backwards placebo effect—a retroactive belief that the pain was not so bad after all. "It's kind of magical that you can alter your memory of pain, and that's what becomes real in the future." (This even works for post-surgical pain, as we discuss in Chapter 5.)

The Power of Parents

Too often, parents feel helpless to make much difference to their child's experience at the doctor's office. But, even as medical professionals take the lead at appointments, parents can actually play an important role. Their efforts to keep their kids calm before, during, and after vaccinations and blood draws can make all the difference in lessening their children's pain.

Rebecca Pillai Riddell, a professor of psychology at York University in Toronto, Canada, researches the influence parents have over their children's responses to pain. In one of her studies, which involved infants and preschoolers during vaccinations, she found that the biggest predictor of a child's distress before a needle was the parent's behavior. If the parent was stressed and anxious before a shot, the child was more likely to be nervous and experience more pain. If, instead, the parent was calm, matter-of-fact, and offered pain-management strategies during injections, the child was more likely to cope well and experience less pain. Dr. Pillai Riddell sums it up: "Parent behavior is a powerful force, and sensitive care-giving before and during vaccinations can reduce a child's distress."[15]

In fact, many studies show that parents have a substantial impact on a child's level of distress, fear, and eventual pain. Researchers have even discovered a few somewhat counterintuitive lessons by studying parent behavior during medical procedures. Meghan Mc-Murtry, an associate professor of psychology, and director of the pediatric pain, health, and communication lab at the University of Guelph, in Canada, has investigated parent behaviors during routine blood draws. The results of her studies are striking. When parents try to reassure their kids with platitudes such as "Don't worry" and "It's okay," the children interpret this as their parents being fearful. This was in part because parents often made worried facial expressions as they said such words. By contrast, when parents in the study calmly discussed other things that were not related to the blood draw (like the poster on the wall), children viewed the parents as less afraid. The results indicate that when a child thinks a

parent is anxious, that only makes the child more afraid. An unruf-
fled parent, it seems, is a key factor in keeping a child calm when
confronted with pain and stress, and thus in reducing the perception
of pain.[16]

Anna and her husband have an acronym for this mindset: KIT,
for *keep it together*. Corny as they know it may be, saying it reminds
them that acting cool, calm, and collected is important for children,
even if you don't feel all that calm on the inside. Anna has also
learned well that even having nothing more than a few fun topics of
conversation in her back pocket as they walk into a doctor's office
can be enough to reduce her children's fear and pain. Talking about
pleasant things in a relaxed tone sends the message that it's an average day and everything is okay.

What if you haven't been aware of these strategies in the past?
Relax. There is always time to turn things around. As Dr. Pillai Riddell says, "It's never too late for a parent to have a positive impact."

Spreading the Word

Pediatric pain researchers have known for years that the pain-relief
techniques outlined in this chapter work, but as Rachel learned the
hard way, the scientific evidence behind the strategies has not yet
made its way into every pediatrician's office. Christine Chambers
at Dalhousie University has pointed out that research typically takes
seventeen years to travel from the research lab to the doctor's
office—and that timeframe is the span of an entire childhood.[17] Not
content to let a whole generation of children miss out on these tools,
Dr. Chambers and several other scientists are reaching out to parents directly.

For example, Dr. Chambers partnered with media influencers and parent groups to launch a social media campaign called "It Doesn't Have to Hurt." Through short videos, blog posts, Facebook, and Twitter, the campaign is educating mothers and fathers about pain-relief techniques and empowering them to use the methods during immunizations and other procedures.

Dr. Cohen at Georgia State University has also found a novel way to connect with parents. His lab is developing and testing a computerized parent-training program called "Bear Essentials," which provides information about what to do and what not to do when preschoolers are getting immunizations. Similarly, the Children's Hospital of Eastern Ontario and the University of Ottawa School of Nursing are collaborating on a "Be Sweet to Babies" initiative, producing videos that show how to ease pain during newborns' blood tests and immunizations.

Another initiative: In 2013, the team at the Children's Hospitals and Clinics of Minnesota implemented its "Children's Comfort Promise," which vows to do everything possible to prevent and treat pain in young patients, and outlines the approach parents can expect practitioners to follow.[18] For instance, kids who undergo a needle procedure at the hospital will be offered topical numbing cream, distraction, their choice of positioning, and a sweet solution (depending on the child's age). "By removing pain from the equation as much as possible, kids see that medical care is here to help them, not hurt them. They're less fearful," says program founder Stefan Friedrichsdorf.

Other practitioners, hospitals, and pediatric institutions also seem to be following suit. Recall, for example, the work of Boston-based ChildKind International (described in Chapter 2), which

Tactics for Parents at the Pediatrician

What can you do to avoid a scenario like the one Rachel faced during her child's immunizations? If the pediatric staff discourages you from using pain-relieving strategies, these tips can help:

· Have a conversation with the pediatrician and ask about her philosophy toward pain management. Ideally, do this before you even choose the practice for your family, so that you'll know what to expect from the practice's protocols surrounding immunizations and other procedures. If you didn't check before signing up with the practice, it's never too late. Remember that it's always your prerogative to ask the doctor questions, and if the answers don't align with your needs, to seek out another practice.

· Take a beat. If, in the moment, the medical staff is moving forward with a painful procedure without allotting time to manage your child's pain, ask the clinician to pause while you consider possible solutions for your child. The odds are good that there is something the practice can do without going outside its protocols to prevent or alleviate the pain. If no solution is possible, it's also okay (in most circumstances) for you to delay the procedure until you have found another practice that is able to do more. It's important that you don't feel pushed into having your child undergo a procedure without proper pain control.

· Don't wait *too* long. While it may make sense to hold off on a procedure until the right protocols are in place, be aware that delaying a necessary procedure might be counterproductive if it means your child spends much more time in a state of anticipatory anxiety.

· Separate your feelings about needle pain from any fears or concerns you may have about immunizations themselves. A desire to avoid pain should not be used as an excuse to forego a vaccination. The life-saving benefits of immunizations far outweigh the sting of a needle poke.

· Deflect damaging messaging. If you hear a clinician telling your child that a shot won't hurt at all, or urging your child to tough it out (something still said particularly to boys, due to the unconscious or conscious bias of some practitioners), counter that message with one of your own. For instance, acknowledge that a shot or needle draw will hurt in the moment, but that it will be over and done quickly. Then, implement the evidence-based pain relief strategies outlined in this chapter. Do your best to distract your child and stay neutral while the clinician does the procedure.

challenges clinicians and hospitals worldwide to improve pain practices, and then recognizes the medical facilities that do so. ChildKind
has developed an accreditation available only to facilities where pain
management for children is demonstrably a priority and explicitly
covered by staff training and protocols. We can only hope that it
eventually becomes standard for every hospital and clinic to earn
certification from ChildKind, thereby ensuring patients and parents
alike that children's pain will be taken seriously.

Chapter 4

Scars from the NICU

*Even when wounds are not visible, they can
leave their marks*

Kyle was born two months premature in April of 1996 in Santa Barbara, California. His mom, Kelly, hadn't experienced any pregnancy complications up to that point, so Kyle's early arrival was a complete surprise to his first-time parents and their doctors. Without any preparation, the new family was thrust into the world of the neonatal intensive care unit (NICU) with its onslaught of bright lights, medical alarms, breathing tubes, and IV lines.

Born at four pounds, five ounces, Kyle wasn't the smallest or sickest baby in the NICU. But that didn't make the experience any less upsetting. "Right after he was born, they whisked him off to the NICU without ever giving him to me; it was traumatic," remembers Kelly. "It was the first time I felt my animal instincts, and thought, 'take me to my baby right now!' And who knows how he felt? He was probably shocked wondering 'where's the love? And what is that poking and prodding me?'"

The unexpectedly early labor meant that, immediately after birth, Kyle wasn't placed on Kelly's chest, where he would have been enveloped by the warmth of her arms, calmed by the smell of her body, and allowed to follow his own instincts to latch and breastfeed. Instead, Kyle was deprived of that human connection from the moment he left the security of the womb. And rather than spending his first month bonding with his mother and father, Kyle's initial exposure to life consisted mostly of lying alone in an incubator where he was hooked up to tubes and given medicine that helped improve his respiration and oxygen levels. He also endured multiple blood draws, was handled by several different hospital staff members each day, and had limited interaction with his parents.

While the medical interventions Kyle received were necessary to keep him alive while his lungs continued to develop, much about the NICU's approach was misguided. Staff wouldn't let Kelly hold or touch Kyle during medical procedures, and they discouraged contact in general—as was then common across the country (and in some NICUs still is). "The nurses would only let me hold him or have skin-to-skin contact with him for five or ten minutes each time because they said any more than that would be overstimulating," says Kelly. "But I truly believe that the noise and constant lights affected him at the time, and later on. I completely believe that for him, as a preemie in the NICU, his nervous system was set on high alarm."

Every Early Poke Counts

Kelly's belief is not just a mother's intuition. Her thinking is backed up by a large body of research on both humans and animals over the past three decades. Experts have found that babies in the NICU typically experience seven to seventeen painful procedures every day.[1] Each of these experiences, ranging from skin pricks to surgeries, impacts how they learn to process pain and stress.[2] Every additional procedure adds to a cumulative effect that can have long-lasting impacts on babies' nervous systems and overall brain development.[3] Studies have shown that among children who spent time in the NICU there is elevated risk of sensory issues, hypersensitivity to pain, developmental delays, anxiety, and other behavioral issues later in life. The greater the number of pain procedures experienced by an infant, the higher that risk rises.[4]

There is, however, an important and hopeful caveat: Research has also shown that certain practices—many of which are simple, safe, non-invasive, and parent-led—can make infants more comfortable during medical procedures, and that using these practices can halt the trajectory of negative outcomes that can otherwise follow an experience of pain, even long after it's over.[5]

How Do Premature Infants Perceive and Show Pain?

Some of the earliest studies on the impact of painful NICU procedures on premature infants were done in the 1980s, when the field of neonatology was still very new.[6] Among the first things scientists evaluated was how these tiny, underdeveloped babies perceive and express pain. Of course, newborns can't talk or point to pictures of frowny faces to indicate their pain levels. And unlike full-term infants, preterm infants often can't react with the typical cues one might expect from a baby. After all, preterm babies haven't had a full thirty-seven to forty weeks in the womb to build all of the neuropathways that connect the peripheral sensory system (where they would sense, say, a needle) to the brain (which would interpret that they are experiencing pain). Nor have they built all the neural connections among different regions of the brain that would enable them to show what they are feeling.

"We take it for granted that it's automatic to react to pain. But it's a mature reaction in the system: the brain has to process a pain signal and then has to mount a response to it, and that involves a lot of steps and neuromessengers that premature infants don't necessarily have," explains Manon Ranger, assistant professor of nursing at the University of British Columbia, in Vancouver, and a pediatric pain researcher at Children's Hospital Research Institute. "But just because infants are not reacting externally, it doesn't mean there is nothing going on in their brain. It's quite the opposite. In fact, in their immature state, premature babies may react more strongly to an input that may not even be painful to an older child or an adult."

Indeed, up until at least thirty-five weeks of gestation, babies' brains are so underdeveloped that they can have trouble differentiating between typically painful stimuli (such as needle pricks) and typically nonpainful stimuli (like diaper changes).[7] The result of this inability to distinguish between various types of touch can mean that even seemingly benign actions, like removing a baby from an incubator to adjust the sheets, can cause pain and stress, which are as real to premature infants as the pain and stress they would experience during a needle injection.

What's more, while older babies are able to regulate themselves after experiencing painful stimuli, premature infants can't yet do so. "Premature babies don't yet have a descending pain pathway, which releases endogenous dopamine, also known as our own natural morphine," says Dr. Ranger. "So they are not capable of dampening their pain response, which is why they feel the pain for longer after experiencing an input."[8]

Taken together, this means that, compared to older babies or adults, the premature infant tends to feel more pain with any stimulus (whether it's a needle prick or IV insertion) and to take much longer to settle back down to a baseline state afterward. And regardless of how premature babies appear to react externally, the daily trauma they experience in the NICU leaves an imprint on the wiring in their brain during a time of significant neural growth—and can shape how they develop.

How do we know what premature infants may be feeling? Researchers have learned how to assess pain in premature infants by studying their reactions (as discussed briefly in Chapter 1). Since the 1980s, scientists including Ruth Grunau, a psychologist and professor of neonatology at the University of British Columbia (and Dr. Ranger's mentor and collaborator), and Celeste Johnston, emeritus professor of nursing at McGill University in Montreal, have established that, while babies cry for many reasons—some related to pain and some not—there are observable facial reactions in premature infants that reliably indicate pain and allow its intensity to be measured.[9]

Still, facial reactions are not foolproof, so researchers have also worked to identify physiological indicators of pain—including increased heart rate, raised blood pressure, lower oxygen saturation, and higher breath rate. Yet because physiological measures can also be influenced by non-pain factors, such as fever and illness, the consensus today is that anyone trying to assess pain in preterm infants should look at the full picture, considering facial reactions, physiological responses, the gestational age of the infant, and the circumstances.

In recent years research on infant pain assessment has become even more nuanced thanks to advances in neuroscience. In some studies, researchers are using electroencephalogram (EEG) and magnetic imaging (MRI) technologies to evaluate how premature infants' brains react during medically necessary procedures. This line of research is especially promising because they have confirmed that a premature infant's observable responses to skin-breaking procedures can be counterintuitive. For example, Dr. Ranger notes that "Some of the babies are so sick or have been so exhausted by interventions that they don't react at all externally. You can see that their brains are reacting, but physically, you would think that they're not in pain because they don't have the energy reserves to react to pain," says Dr. Ranger.

Based on all that she has learned, Dr. Ranger advises hospital staff and parents to make a basic assumption: "Anything that would be painful to you, will be painful to them, and perhaps even more so." Keeping this in mind helps to reinforce the importance of preventing that pain or discomfort whenever possible. So, if your child is in the NICU, be sure to ask what measures staff are taking to relieve pain—and learn the helpful strategies outlined below, which you may be able to implement with them. This will not only make a baby's immediate experience easier, it may also reduce the life-long effects of early painful exposures.[10]

Simple and Safe Parent-Led Pain Management

Analgesics and topical anesthetics (such as numbing creams) are of course important medications to prevent pain in preterm infants. But there are some instances when they may not be appropriate. Fortunately, some of the most effective pain management techniques are natural, low-cost, and parent-centered. The best example is skin-to-skin contact—also called kangaroo care—which is the practice of placing a baby on the bare chest of the mother or other loved one so that one's flesh is in full contact with the other's, with the two often covered by a blanket. Studies have found that skin-to-skin contact not only promotes an infant's general well-being, it also significantly reduces the pain response and soothes the nervous system of an infant undergoing a medical procedure.[11] Even more ideal for these purposes is to add in nursing, which provides a complete sensory and physiological experience, and has been shown to be the most effective in reducing pain. But if breastfeeding is not possible (for instance, a baby in the NICU may not have learned to latch to the breast), it is helpful to provide a pacifier or feed the infant breast milk or formula from a bottle or dropper while providing skin-to-skin contact.

"Historically, mothers have always been crucial to infant survival and well-being but they are not always involved in critical care settings," says Marsha Campbell-Yeo, a neonatal nurse and clinical scientist at the Centre for Pediatric Pain Research at IWK Health Centre, and a professor of nursing at Dalhousie University. "But through our research we've found that skin-to-skin contact with mothers—and other caregivers—has powerful benefits and can significantly reduce pain responses in preterm and full-term infants undergoing a painful procedure." Dr. Campell-Yeo and her colleagues recognize how much a caregiver's touch matters: "It lessens how much the baby feels in response to pain, it stabilizes their heart rate and oxygen levels, and helps them recover from the pain faster."[12]

Dr. Campbell-Yeo also notes that there are payoffs to kangaroo care for parents, as well. The comforting interaction brings parents and babies closer, it triggers the release of oxytocin (the "love hormone" that facilitates bonding), and helps parents feel more confident and in control during what is often an upsetting time. There are few things more distressing than seeing your baby in pain and being forced to stand back and watch, feeling helpless to alleviate their suffering. Skin-to-skin contact is proof that parents can make a difference.

Research led by Dr. Campbell-Yeo and Dr. Johnston finds that, to get the most out of kangaroo care or breastfeeding, skin-to-skin contact should start just before a painful procedure (between two and fifteen minutes in advance) and, if possible, continue until the procedure is over and the baby has recovered from the pain and stress. But even if kangaroo care or breastfeeding cannot be done during the procedure, there are still significant pain-reducing benefits to providing either strategy for two to fifteen minutes before a procedure.

Sugar Benefits and Drawbacks

Another widely used tactic to reduce premature infants' pain is to give them a sucrose solution (sugar water) starting about two minutes before and ideally, continuing during a medical procedure. Dr. Campbell-Yeo explains that the practice of giving sucrose evolved in the 1980s, when clinicians began recognizing the importance of treating pain in premature infants yet found that giving repeated doses of opioids had negative side effects. "More medication is not always better, and it was in that context that we recognized the need to find a balance between exposing tiny babies to medications and also blocking their pain," says Dr. Campbell-Yeo. "In looking for opioid sparing options, that brought forth a lot of the work around nonpharmacologic interventions."

The sweet-tasting liquid was seen as an alternative to pain-relieving drugs for minor procedures such as heel pricks, and studies found that when sucrose was given just before a procedure involving a needle, it appeared to quiet fussy babies and calm their reactions.[13] As a result, giving infants sucrose (usually via a dropper of sugar water) became the gold standard in NICUs. But as with standard medications, researchers have discovered that more sucrose is not necessarily better, and there may be some unintended consequences of giving too many doses of sucrose per day.

"What's happened is that NICU staff members may give sucrose to babies ten times a day, during each procedure, without acknowledging that sucrose is an artificial substance," says Dr. Ranger, "and we don't know how repeated doses of sucrose every day may affect a developing brain long-term." While the amount of sugar may seem small, it can add up, especially when given to a tiny infant. "Of course *not* treating pain is worse than giving sucrose," Dr. Ranger emphasizes, "but our research in mice has found that when sucrose is given repeatedly, this impacts the immature brain, and later in life, this can affect multiple important brain structures, like the hippocampus, which is related to memory."[14]

While it's not entirely clear if sucrose works on pain pathways, stress pathways, or both, the potentially negative effects of giving too much sucrose to preterm infants has led some NICUs, including the hospitals where Dr. Ranger works, to do away with administering sugar water during medical procedures. Other hospitals continue to use sucrose to reduce needle-related pain, but at the hospital where Dr. Campbell-Yeo works, for instance, the revised message to NICU staff members and parents is that other pain-relieving interventions, such as skin-to-skin contact, are preferred and should be used first. "We now know that skin-to-skin contact or breastfeeding is at least as effective as giving sucrose, if not more effective," says Dr. Campbell-Yeo. "That's not to say anything bad about sweet taste, but it is to say that parents are our most underutilized resource in the NICU."

Additional Pain-Relieving NICU Practices

There are other second-tier ways that parents and hospital staff can alleviate the stress and pain of medical procedures in the NICU. Though not as effective as the first-tier methods of skin-to-skin contact, breastfeeding, sucrose, and numbing cream, these methods offer some comfort; and implementing them during a medical procedure is much better than offering no pain control. Additionally, when they are used together with frontline interventions, they enhance the effects.

These second-tier pain-relieving techniques include non-nutritive sucking (such as sucking on a pacifier); facilitated tucking (where the hands of a parent or nurse are placed around the baby's limbs, head, or both to provide comfort); swaddling; music; and maternal smell (allowing a baby who cannot be near their mother to smell a piece of the mother's clothing). It is inevitable in a NICU that babies sometimes need a medical intervention when a parent is not at hand. These interventions can be particularly useful in such instances.

On the horizon, there may soon be another option: under development now is a robotic platform that's placed inside an incubator, called the Calmer, which simulates the sound of a mother's heartbeat, the subtle up-and-down movements of her breathing, and her skin-like feel. Created by Liisa Holsti, an associate professor of occupational science and occupational therapy at the University of British Columbia, the device is intended to serve as "backup" skin-to-skin contact when a family member can't be present for a medical procedure. Early research has shown that this multi-sensory intervention works as well as standard care when used at least fifteen minutes before a painful procedure, during it, and for about five minutes afterward. "The device helps calm babies down more quickly and they return to their baseline faster, and it was just as effective at reducing pain reactions in the NICU as was facilitated tucking," says Dr. Ranger, who was involved in the device's clinical trials.

The study authors also found that the Calmer relieved some of the stress that mothers felt when they couldn't be in the NICU to comfort their babies during a procedure. "The idea is not to replace mothers," says Dr. Ranger. "But parents told us that they were happy to know that, if they couldn't be there with their baby, then there was something that could be done to help them through a procedure."[15]

Missed Opportunities for Pain Relief

Despite the studies showing how preterm babies experience pain and how it can be managed, many NICUs have yet to fully take advantage of pain-relieving interventions, often due to a lack of awareness of this growing body of research. "When I started in the NICU, there was really little or no attention paid to pain, because the whole concept was that babies didn't feel or remember pain—and we have come a very long way since then," says Dr. Campbell-Yeo. But even in the most advanced NICUs, she says, it is still often true that clinicians deprioritize pain management. Institutionalized systems tend not to change quickly.

"Healthcare providers really do want to do the best job and reduce harm in their patients. But sometimes, especially in a critical care setting, they think the procedural task is more important than managing the pain—when in fact that is true only in very few cases," says Dr. Campbell-Yeo. "The majority of babies could wait for five minutes to get the pain-relieving medication before the procedure is done; or the clinician could wait for the mother to implement kangaroo care before starting the IV line or whatever the task may be."

But old habits die hard, and the result is often very little extra time spent in the service of making the baby more comfortable in the short term and improving the baby's health and development later in life.

Karen, a former neonatal nurse, has seen this variability in NICUs as both a staff member and as a mother whose baby was in the NICU. She worked in the NICU at Brigham and Women's Hospital in Boston in the late 1980s and was trained in the philosophy of Heidelise Als, a professor of psychology and director of neurobehavioral infant and child studies at Harvard Medical School. Dr. Als was at the forefront of assessing and managing neonatal pain when she developed the Newborn Individualized Developmental Care and Assessment Program (NIDCAP), which has since been implemented in NICUs around the world.[16]

"We were taught that the sights and sounds of the NICU were overwhelming to the infants and our job was to minimize the traumatic exposures these infants had each day," says Karen. To that end, the NICU where Karen worked had ambient lighting, the nurses put blankets over the isolettes to create a womb-like environment, and the staff grouped procedures together whenever they could so that the infants didn't have to endure the stress of extra disruptions.

"At Brigham, the nurses were really empowered. We had a primary care model where one nurse would work with the same baby every day, and there were times you had to act like a policeman to guard your baby from a resident or attending physician who attempted to disturb the baby for an intervention that was not necessary at that time," says Karen. "Some of the doctors thought we were slowing them down, but many of the doctors jumped on the bandwagon and saw the benefits of this approach for the babies and parents."

Unfortunately, for Karen, when her son Zach was born in 1995 and needed to spend two weeks in a NICU in New Jersey, the staff there did not ascribe to the NIDCAP philosophy or anything similar. Zach was born full-term, but during labor he breathed in meconium (fetal stool). Given the risk of severe complications, this required that he be treated in the NICU. But as far as Karen was told, there was no pain management when Zach received skin-breaking procedures, and they were so distressing to his system that his lungs collapsed during two separate blood draws. "I felt like every time they touched him, they would stick him and he would pop a lung," she remembers.

To reinflate Zach's lungs, the staff had to insert chest tubes, and Karen was never told if there was any pain management during those procedures. "Imagine someone sticking a tube all the way through your ribs into your lungs with no pain control," says Karen. "I kept saying, 'leave him alone,' and I wanted to be a mom first, not a NICU nurse, but when I saw they were not covering the babies from light, or minimizing the sounds, and they weren't grouping the medical interventions together, I felt I needed to speak up for my baby."

Even with her professional nursing background and experience advocating for fragile babies in the NICU, Karen found it extremely difficult to advocate for her own son. She had just given birth, she was exhausted and terrified, and she felt pushed aside in the midst of life-or-death decisions about her infant's health. "They didn't give me the option of skin-to-skin care and when I told the staff not to touch my baby, I could tell I got their child abuse or neglect sirens going, because they kept questioning me about why I didn't want certain interventions," she says.

In 2000, in Buffalo, New York, another mother didn't push back on any particular interventions when her identical twin sons were born at thirty-one weeks and placed in the NICU. Tina, like Karen in New Jersey and Kelly in California, remembers scant talk of pain management in the month and a half her babies were in the hospital. Vincent was five pounds, seven ounces and Jacob was three pounds, thirteen ounces, and both boys were placed in incubators and given IV lines and breathing tubes. Vincent also needed extensive blood transfusions, a process that Tina remembers looked horrifying. "He was strapped down, bruised, not fully diapered or covered, and he was all hooked up to wires with an IV in his navel, head, and in a vein in his arm," says Tina.

The new mom wasn't able to hold Jacob until he was three days old, and couldn't touch or hold Vincent until he was twelve days old. "You wonder what the developmental implications of that are, sensory-wise," says Tina, who is a pediatric speech therapist and reading specialist. "That's a long time to be strapped to a bunch of wires, even though obviously they needed it."

To this day, Tina believes that her sons' early life experiences in the NICU have something to do with the developmental delays they had to overcome. Both required speech therapy for several years to address severely delayed speech, and occupational therapy to improve their gross motor development. The boys also needed extra help with reading, executive functioning, and emotional growth throughout their schooling. "They also always needed extra sensory stimulation in order to regulate their nervous systems," remembers Tina. It likely didn't settle their nerves that even after their time in the NICU, for the first six months they were home, they wore oxygen monitors twenty-four hours a day that would often detach and trigger shrill alarms.

Tina's belief that a NICU experience can affect a child's development is backed up by research. To be sure, many factors can

contribute to developmental delays in infants who are born premature, including genetics and underlying neurological differences, but
studies show that babies treated in the NICU have a significantly
increased risk of developing cognitive and physical delays. Estimates
show that half of NICU graduates with low birth weights will experience developmental or learning disabilities, and about one in
ten will have social difficulties, inattention, or permanent motor
problems.[17]

Kelly's son, who arrived two months early in California in 1996,
also showed significant sensory-seeking behavior throughout his
childhood. "He definitely struggled as a younger kid. He was my
high-intensity baby, and it was very clear that his nervous system
needed more care than his younger sister's did," says Kelly. "He always needed a lot more calming touch, and we did occupational
therapy to help with sensory issues and his coordination." Thinking
back on their time in the NICU, Kelly says, "it never occurred to me
to ask for pain management even when I watched the blood draws
and saw him flinch. It was painful, clearly; and we also had to give
him medication that would make him cringe and vomit. I just assumed there was no other choice."

Even Kelly's last experience in the NICU involved a lack of pain
management. "The staff recommended we do a circumcision on our
last day in the NICU before sending us home. I asked if I could go
with my son and they said, 'no, no.' Looking back on it now, I would
not have done the circumcision then; I was delirious," she says. When
the nurse brought Kelly's son back to her, there was a large scratch
on his face, and the nurse said the baby had scratched himself during
the circumcision. "I remember thinking he must have been in pain
if he scratched his face so badly, and I thought, why do we do this?
What is going on?" The nurses all said, 'don't worry, babies don't

remember this.' But later, as we went to occupational therapy, I thought, 'this kid remembers this. His body remembers all of this, without a doubt.'"

Again, Kelly's instincts were right. Groundbreaking research led by Anna Taddio and published in *The Lancet* in 1997, one year after Kelly's son was born, demonstrated that babies who don't receive a topical anesthetic (a numbing cream) during circumcision show increased pain responses during vaccinations at four and six months compared to babies who either do receive an anesthetic during circumcision or are not circumcised. In short, painful experiences during infancy can have far-reaching effects. Babies may not consciously remember early painful procedures, but their nervous systems certainly do.[18]

Progress on NICU Pain Protocols

Today, most major hospitals have physicians who specialize in pain management, and NICUs are consistently working toward improving their pain-reducing protocols.[19] But parents shouldn't assume that every NICU is up to date on the latest pain management measures. Given how long it takes for research to be disseminated and put into practice, there are always some NICUs at the forefront of pain management and others that are not. "I would say that about 50 percent of babies even in North America go through needle-related pain or tissue-breaking pain, and don't get pain control," says Dr. Campbell-Yeo.

To improve those odds, Dr. Campbell-Yeo has studied why skin-to-skin contact isn't implemented in certain situations. Her research reveals that, 35 percent of the time, parents aren't present when a medical procedure is performed on an infant in the NICU.[20] How can parents facilitate pain management if they're not given the opportunity to participate in their infants' care? The answer, according to Dr. Campbell-Yeo and many other pediatric pain experts, is that parents should be educated about their invaluable role in the NICU from the get-go. She is in the process of developing an online learning platform for families that will teach them how to soothe and advocate for their babies in the NICU, and how best to participate in their overall care.[21]

Dr. Campbell-Yeo and one of her PhD students, Brianna Richardson, are also developing an online platform called Parenting Pain Away, designed to teach pregnant moms ways to reduce pain in healthy babies after birth. "We know most babies receive an intramuscular injection and a metabolic blood test screening shortly after birth, and those procedures should be done along with skin-to-skin contact or when breastfeeding," says Dr. Campbell-Yeo. Whether or not a baby is in the NICU, all early exposures to painful medical procedures are opportunities to shape a baby's nervous system for the better.

Fortunately for families today, the messages about pain control and parent involvement seem to be getting out, with life-changing impact. Calvin and his wife are New York City residents whose son Isaac was born in 2016 with what is called a giant omphalocele, a birth defect by which the intestines grow outside the abdomen. Isaac spent the first fourteen months of his life in the hospital and went through multiple surgeries involving his abdomen and heart. The ordeal was harrowing, but his parents discovered early on how to comfort their son and be part of his care. "We learned quickly that the best way to help Isaac was to be informed and to be his advocates," says Calvin. "As the only constants in his life in the middle of many different clinicians, we took really detailed notes, and we were there to keep him as calm as possible during blood draws and other procedures."

The two first-time parents were as hands-on as they could be, literally and figuratively. "One of us would always hold one of Isaac's arms while a nurse would be doing a medical procedure so at least a familiar hand would be holding him rather than a gloved hand of the nurse," Calvin says. They also eventually learned to handle much of the maintenance of the medical equipment themselves, like changing their son's tracheostomy tube (the breathing tube inserted in his neck). "There really wasn't anything that my wife and I didn't do, and I think it helped us manage his pain and communicate with him better," says Calvin.

Jackie, of Fort Meyers, Florida, also learned how to soothe her newborn triplets when they spent seven weeks in the NICU in 2019, and she was emboldened to do so by the NICU staff. "They were all less than three pounds and we couldn't take them out of the incubator for four days after they were born, but the nurses taught us how to do 'hand hugs' [the facilitated tucking described above], which was a way for us to touch them that was calming and soothing rather than overstimulating."

The NICU where the triplets stayed had private rooms with low lights and muted TVs, which required headphones, so that the noise and lights around the infants didn't create sensory overload. "The staff explained that so much of the touch preemies get in the NICU is not positive touch, so they empowered us to do what we could—and taught us how to hold and touch them in calming ways even when somebody was changing their diaper, or taking their temperature," says Jackie. The nurses also encouraged both Jackie and her husband to do kangaroo care, and taught them how to gently massage their infants to enhance their range of motion, improve their

Minimizing Your Baby's Pain in the NICU

The NICU can seem like a realm of experts where parents have no authority, but the following tips can help you make a big difference to your baby's care.*

- Ask the NICU staff about their pain assessment and management protocols, and tell them clearly that you would like your baby's pain to be prevented or managed for every potentially painful procedure. Also, consider asking the staff to group your baby's procedures together, when possible, to minimize the amount of times she is disturbed.

- Start kangaroo care and skin-to-skin contact (such holding your baby's hand) as soon as possible. It can be difficult and nerve-wracking to hold very small babies because they are extremely fragile. But as soon as you're comfortable, this tactile connection can be a vital part of your baby's pain management. And moms are not the only ones who can provide this comfort; dads and other loved ones can do kangaroo care, too.

- In addition to kangaroo care, there are nonpharmacologic strategies to help alleviate your infant's pain during brief procedures such as needlesticks. Try breastfeeding (bottle-feeding may also help), pacifier use, tucking or swaddling, or oral sucrose—and use more than one of these, if possible.

- For prolonged painful procedures (for example, a lumbar puncture or catheter insertion), ask the NICU staff to give your baby pain medication. These types of extended skin-breaking procedures should include topical anesthetics and possibly a low dose of systemic medication such as an opioid.

- If your baby develops a painful condition such as necrotizing enterocolitis (NEC)—an inflammation of the intestines that sometimes affects premature infants—talk with your child's care team to learn about the pain medications that are being administered. Be aware that opioid infusions are often recommended in these cases.

- Don't hesitate to alert the NICU staff if you notice a change in how your baby is behaving or responding. Often, parents are the first ones to notice that their baby is in pain.

- Keep in mind that you can advocate for your baby even when you can't be in the NICU. Many families are not able to have a parent present in the hospital every day.† But NICUs often have volunteers available to hold babies. If you're interested in this option for your baby, let the staff know.

---

* Anand, "Prevention and Treatment of Neonatal Pain," UpToDate, updated May 28, 2021.

† S. N. Saxton, B. L. Walker, and D. Dukhovny, "Parents Matter: Examination of Family Presence in the Neonatal Intensive Care Unit," *American Journal of Perinatology* 38, no. 10 (2021): 1023–1030.

sensory development, and aid their digestive system. "Our involvement really allowed us, the parents, to be the comfort givers," says Jackie.

Whether the NICU environment is state-of-the-art or behind the times, for so many parents, the simple act of being with their babies, touching them, and holding them whenever possible can provide comfort not just for the infants in the hospital but also for the parents. The overall result is calmer, happier, and healthier families.

Of course, many parents are not able to take time away from work or from taking care of their other children to be with their infants in the NICU at all times, especially when the stay is long or when the baby needs specialized care in a hospital far from home. In these cases, nurses and hospital volunteers can fill in and offer calming touch and soothing interventions. Parents should feel empowered to ask the NICU staff to ensure that pain-reducing measures are taken when needed. Even from afar, parents can advocate for their child's pain management.

The experience of giving birth and caring for a newborn is physically and emotionally exhausting (most obviously for mothers, but

also for their partners), and the stress of having an infant who requires immediate medical attention is an enormous weight for parents to bear. "It took me a long time to process the trauma of my
son's preemiehood," says Kelly, whose son Kyle is now in law school.
"He grew into a strong, capable adult," she says. But for much of
his life, Kelly couldn't shake the feeling that Kyle was fragile and
needed protecting. Managing pain well—and empowering parents
to be a part of the process—is one clear way to minimize the stress
of the NICU for families and give children's nervous systems the best
possible support for development.

Chapter 5

Surgeries, Minor Medical Procedures, and Hospital Visits

*How to prepare for these, and
how kids remember them*

It is increasingly common that children experience the hospital setting. Each year, about five million children in the United States undergo surgeries and other medical procedures that require anesthesia. These include major inpatient surgeries (for example, spinal fusion), minor outpatient surgeries (for example, tonsillectomies and ear tube placements), and other procedures requiring sedation (for example, colonoscopies and lumbar punctures). Because of advances in medical technology and changes in payment arrangements and insurance, this number has steadily grown over the past decade.[1] The number of pediatric procedures requiring anesthesia has also grown in Europe.[2] What's more, many millions of children with chronic illnesses and short-term conditions regularly undergo blood draws, IV insertions, injections, and stitches as part of their care. Thus, a significant number of children find themselves in hospitals, urgent care facilities, and surgical centers facing inherently painful procedures that are typically scary for them and stressful for their parents.

While some pain from surgeries and procedures is inevitable, there is a lot that providers and parents can do to minimize it, not all of which is always implemented. We've progressed exponentially since the days of Jeffrey Lawson's tragic surgery in the 1980s, but we can still do better. Fortunately, researchers continue to refine pain-relieving strategies for children undergoing medical procedures, and parents continue to champion them.

Wendy's Story: Taking Control

Wendy, a seventeen-year old who lives outside of Boston, learned at a very young age about the pain of surgeries and medical procedures. When she was three years old she contracted *Escherichia coli* (*E. coli*), a bacterial infection, and went from being a healthy, carefree preschooler to being a full-time patient in the hospital for weeks on end. In Wendy's case, the *E. coli* infection led to a condition called hemolytic uremic syndrome (HUS), which triggered a complex set of medical problems including heart failure, seizures, and damage to her intestines, pancreas, and kidneys. By the time Wendy was five years old, she'd been on a ventilator many times, she'd had several surgeries to remove parts of her intestines, she'd undergone a kidney transplant, and the damage to her pancreas had caused her to become diabetic and dependent on external insulin.

Wendy's mother, Darcy, describes those early years—filled with frequent trips to the emergency department and more than two hundred days in the hospital—as terrifying and overwhelming. But in the next breath, she explains that she and her family have also learned a great deal about how to make it through medical procedures, prolonged hospital stays, and the demands that come with living with a chronic illness.

Over the years, Wendy, who Darcy calls her "brave, fragile warrior," has become an expert in managing her fear and pain. "When I was little, and I'd get blood work done, I used to need five or six people holding me down because I was so afraid of needles, but I've calmed down a lot since then," says Wendy. "I got comfortable with needles going into me, because I had to do it so many times." One thing that helped her get to that point was her parents' resolve to give her as much control over medical situations—and her own body—as they could. This began with small choices: which finger to prick to test her blood sugar, which snack to eat if her blood sugar was low. Wendy chose the meal she'd eat the night before a surgery, the scent of the anesthesia mask she would get, and the stuffed animal she would bring with her to the hospital (Teddy, every time).

As Wendy grew older, "we tried to give her more control and more choice," says Darcy. Wendy, now in high school, still has health issues and, as a transplant survivor, is immunocompromised, so it's not uncommon for her to end up in the emergency department with an infection. "She still has hurdles, she is still diabetic, she still takes medication daily, and worries about infections, and has some dietary restrictions—but she doesn't let it hold her back," explains Darcy, who points out that Wendy now swims competitively, runs track, and is on a soccer team. No doubt in part because of the independence Wendy's parents gave her, she's also figured out her own ways of doing things: "When my IV hurts, I ask for a warm pack because the fluid in the IV is cold. It doesn't really numb the pain but it just warms it up so my hand feels better," says Wendy. "And sometimes you have to flush the IV and I like to do it myself. The nurse would do it fast but it feels better to go slow, and I also want to control it. I like being in control of the things that go into my own body." Being in charge of parts of their experience can be crucial for children in a hospital setting, particularly because so many other aspects of their treatment and their lives are beyond their control.

Learning What to Expect

Wendy and Darcy even figured out a way to help other kids feel more in control and less scared at the hospital. They scripted and helped produce an animated video, narrated by Wendy, that explains what kids will see and do when they go to the emergency department.[3] The project, which was conceived by Wendy and Darcy and developed with a team at Boston's MassGeneral Hospital for Children, is now available on the hospital's website. In the video, the animated Wendy (in a dark pink hoodie and a bright green hat) gives a virtual tour of the emergency department, tells kids about the nurses and doctors they might meet, and shows typical procedures children may experience. The goal, says Darcy, is to give kids information in terms they can grasp when they arrive at the hospital afraid and in pain. "If you think about it, every time you go on an airplane, you get instructions on what is going to happen during the flight, including what might happen in an emergency," says Darcy. "Wouldn't you feel better if you got some instruction or information while you were waiting to be seen in the hospital?"

Wendy and Darcy's idea is spot on. Providing kid-friendly information about the hospital is one of the approaches that researchers have found to be effective in reducing preoperative anxiety in children. Many other hospitals also offer age-appropriate surgical-prep programs, whether through video tours, in-person visits, or picture books. By giving young patients a visual narrative of what to expect, all these forms of educational preparation lessen kids' fear of the unknown.[4]

Keeping Kids Calm Prior to Surgery

While reducing stress and fear prior to medical procedures is an important goal on its own, it actually serves a dual purpose: research shows that when children experience less anxiety before surgery, they tend to have less post-operative pain and require less pain medication in the days after surgery.[5] Once again, we see how stress and fear are intricately tied to the perception of pain. One part of the surgery process that scientists and clinicians have focused on improving over the years is the crucial period of induction, when anesthesia is being administered and the child is making the mind-altering transition from being awake to being unconscious.

Keep in mind that an operating room can look like a scary place, particularly for children who may not fully understand why they are there or what's going to happen to them. With its bright lights, sterile walls, beeping machines, and array of masked adults bustling about, the room does not inspire calm. Therefore, the pivotal moments of induction, when the anesthesia mask is being placed on the face, can be traumatic for children and stressful for parents—and easing anxiety during this time can dramatically improve the surgical experience.

Currently, evidence suggests that distraction—a seemingly simple solution—is one of the best ways to calm children during induction. Researchers have found that letting kids play video games before induction, giving kids a video to watch during induction, and using hypnosis techniques are all effective distraction approaches pre-surgery.[6] Remarkably, in some instances, they can be just as effective in calming children as the medication that's typically given prior to surgery to induce drowsiness and relaxation.[7] Distraction methods can also have lasting effects. In studies, children who were distracted and soothed with video games or hypnosis prior to surgery had fewer behavioral problems during the week after surgery.

In one recent study, a group of children ranging from six to twelve years old were taught a relaxation-guided imagery technique an hour before their surgery, while another group of children received standard pre-operative care. The training, which took a mere fifteen minutes, taught the children how to relax their muscles from the tip of their toes to the top of their head, and visualize a favorite place or experience while remembering the relaxing sensations associated with it (for example, by thinking back to a family visit to the beach, and imagining the feel of the sand between their toes, the smell of the sea air, and the caress of a light breeze on their arms). The children were then prompted to repeat the exercise as they were about to go into surgery. The researchers found that the kids who did the relaxation technique had significantly less anxiety at induction *and* less pain after surgery than the children who didn't learn the technique.[8]

Note that parents don't have to be experts in guided imagery techniques to help their kids benefit from these strategies. There are apps available to lead children through relaxation exercises, and kids can do them on their own or with their parents' assistance. Also, many hospitals have certified professionals on staff known as child life specialists, whose job it is to help kids cope in medical settings. These specialists are trained to lessen kids' stress during medical procedures and prior to surgery by offering distractions (such as videos, bubbles, squeeze balls, and games), breathing exercises (which might include blowing pinwheels), and guided imagery. Some even teach children how to soothe themselves.

Evidence also shows that the overall pre-surgical environment can make a big difference in how much anxiety and pain children experience. We know this in part because of research led by Zeev Kain, a pediatric anesthesiologist and executive director of the Center on Stress and Health at the University of California at Irvine. Much of what we know about minimizing children's stress and fear surrounding surgery is informed by his work. In an early study, he looked at how the typical noisy, busy, and bright hospital setting affects children undergoing surgery. Children in this study were randomly assigned to two groups, with the first (the high sensory stimuli group) experiencing a standard preoperative environment and the second (the low sensory stimuli group) experiencing a more soothing atmosphere. Specifically, the latter were placed in a room with dim lighting and classical music playing softly, and each was cared for by just one provider. The children in the low sensory stimuli group were significantly less anxious and more cooperative during the induction period.[9] While it has since been widely established that a calming preoperative environment can soothe children and improve their outcomes, not all hospitals offer this or are equipped to cater to children's particular needs. Parents would be wise to ask hospital staff in advance about the preoperative environment, and request child focused interventions when possible. (Suggestions on preparing a child for surgery and easing the recovery period are provided at the end of this chapter.)

Dr. Kain has also studied whether it's helpful for children to have a parent in the operating room during induction. What he found, surprisingly, is that simply having a parent present at induction is not enough to reduce a child's anxiety or improve cooperation. After all, some parents feel anxious watching their child go into surgery and may not be in a state of mind to effectively calm their child.[10] For this reason, it's important for parents to talk with the hospital staff before surgery to find out if they will be allowed in the operating room prior to the procedure, and if so, how they can be most helpful in that setting. Some hospitals offer resources to educate parents on ways to make their presence in the room most supportive.

The Role of Memory

In Chapter 3, we talked about how a child's memory of a vaccination can influence subsequent pain responses. The same principle applies when children undergo surgeries and other painful medical procedures. Scientists have even shown that, not only do children remember surgical or procedural pain later in life, those memories can affect how they later respond to pain medications. Research has demonstrated that children who did not receive adequate pain treatment during medical procedures are more likely than children who did receive appropriate pain control to require higher levels of pain medication for subsequent painful procedures.[11] "The notion that children can't remember has led to a lot of suffering," says Melanie Noel, an associate professor of psychology at the University of Calgary. She is quick to add that we know better now—and that a child's recollection of an experience can be reshaped. "Kids memories are so suggestible that just the way adults talk to kids about these experiences can actually change the memory of it and influence how they anticipate pain in the future."

In a recent study, Dr. Noel and her team checked in with young tonsillectomy patients at two points, assessing the kids' pain levels right after surgeries, and meeting with them and their parents two weeks later. For the second meeting, parents were instructed to talk as they normally would with their child about the surgery, and after some time in conversation the kids were asked to recall how much pain they had felt right after the surgery. Amazingly, when the parents used more positive language and did not focus on the painful parts of the experience, the kids remembered the pain after the surgery as less severe than they had originally rated it. These children had developed more positive memories than the kids whose conversations with their parents had focused more on the pain.[12] The narratives we tell ourselves, and in turn, the narratives we remember, can set the stage for our future responses to painful procedures.

Dr. Noel emphasizes that it is vital that children's pain be effectively managed during procedures and surgeries in the first place, but she is also hopeful about harnessing the power of memories to ease children's subsequent pain. "We've shown that you can teach parents in fifteen minutes how to talk to their kids and to actually get their kids to remember surgery in a positive way," says Dr. Noel. "Just with discussions afterwards, you can reframe how children are going to remember the experience for the rest of their lives."

Dr. Noel's advice for parents? As discussed in Chapter 3, talk about painful events or experiences soon after they've happened, but don't evoke the pain sensations by repeatedly using words like *pain, ouch,* and *hurt.* Instead, focus on other aspects of the experience, like the nice nurse who arrived with a popsicle after surgery, or the cool fish tank in the lobby. She also suggests that parents talk about any strategies kids used to promote their own calm before, during, or after the procedure. Affirming these can help build children's confidence in their abilities to handle such experiences in general. For instance, you might point out that your child did a great job of taking deep breaths during a blood draw or focusing on a video game while getting an IV inserted. Offering kudos and reminding kids of techniques they have used to improve their own experience can be particularly important for children with chronic medical conditions, who have to undergo repeated painful procedures.

Stopping Persistent Post-Surgical Pain

While pediatric anesthesiologists over the past decades have vastly improved the management of children's pain during surgery, scientists are still learning how to reduce pain that persists *after* major surgeries. Research led by Jennifer Rabbitts, a pediatric anesthesiologist at the Seattle Children's Hospital and associate professor at the University of Washington, has found that about 20 percent of children still have some pain twelve months after major surgical procedures, such as spinal fusions.[13]

According to Dr. Rabbitts, whose research focuses on surgical pain in adolescents, physicians are starting to use regional anesthetics more frequently during surgery (in both adults and children) in addition to general anesthesia to guard against unrelenting post-surgical pain. This approach involves injecting local anesthetics near a cluster of nerves to numb the area of the body where the surgery is focused. "For kids, the regional block will usually be done after they are asleep but before the procedure starts," says Dr. Rabbitts. "The goal is for pain relief after the surgery." She notes that this approach can be very effective in minimizing short-term pain after surgery, which may also lead to reduced long-term pain.

Preventing intractable pain also reduces the need for high levels of opioid medications post-surgery. Dr. Rabbitts explains that opioids (which block pain by attaching to receptors in the central nervous system and brain) are indeed frequently necessary for children during surgery, and often afterward. But because these medications have severe side effects—including respiratory problems, drowsiness, nausea, and the risk of addiction—they should be used only when needed. "Nationally, there has been a lot of concern about exposing children to opioids, and a big focus on reducing that, but in many instances, we haven't offered something else," says Dr. Rabbits. This has created confusion among both clinicians and parents about which pain medications should be prescribed to children after surgery.

Recent evidence also shows that the prescription of opioids after outpatient surgeries, such as tonsillectomies, is not associated with reduced complications or fewer return visits for pain or dehydration; rather, opioids increase the likelihood of constipation following the surgery.[14] This suggests that opioids are not the best way to manage pain after surgery, especially when used on their own. Fortunately, there are new clinical guidelines for prescribing opioids to children after surgery.[15] There is also a growing movement (and new recommendations for specific surgeries like tonsillectomies) for physicians to prescribe non-opioid pain relievers along with opioid medication during and after surgery. It has been shown that the addition of acetaminophen (Tylenol) or a non-steroidal anti-inflammatory drug (NSAID) such as ibuprofen (Advil) reduces the amount of opioids needed to adequately manage children's pain.[16] (For more on opioids, see Chapter 10.)

Still, families should not have unreasonable expectations about how children will feel after surgery. "We can't take away all the pain with our pain treatments. It's not realistic to think that post-operative pain can be treated to a zero. So if kids have been told 'don't worry, we'll treat all your pain,' it can be hard to experience pain post-op," says Dr. Rabbitts. "There is a need to prepare them for what's realistic after surgery and what's safe."

There are, of course, also non-pharmacologic ways to reduce post-surgical pain. Just as it matters to reduce kids' anxiety before surgery, it's also vital to ensure they get adequate sleep beforehand. Research led by Dr. Rabbitts found that, compared to kids who got sufficient sleep each night, adolescents who had shorter durations of sleep in the week before surgery had higher pain intensity two weeks after surgery. This strong correlation between sleep and pain indicates that getting enough rest before a surgical procedure could make a big difference in a child's recovery.

How can parents motivate their kids to get enough sleep and take an active part in their pre-surgery health? Given that many teenagers resist their parents' proddings in an effort to assert their independence, you might consider outsourcing this task to a smart phone application. Dr. Rabbitts and her team have developed an app for young people to use both before and after surgery that teaches them psychological and behavioral strategies (like deep breathing) proven to reduce anxiety and pain. Designed to put pain-relieving tools in kids' hands from the get-go, the app also has the benefit of building what is known as pain self-efficacy—a confidence in one's ability to manage pain that research shows is related to better recovery from pain after surgery.[17] (Recall Wendy's understanding that, the more control she had over her own body and her own care, the better she felt.) Dr. Rabbitts and her team hope to see the app's effectiveness proved in clinical trials, and then to make it broadly available to teens and parents. In the wake of the Covid-19 pandemic, which caused many clinicians and patients to move away from in-person appointments and become more comfortable with digital options, it is easy to imagine this app appealing to many users.

Finally, coaching parents prior to their child's surgery is key. "We need to help parents be prepared to get themselves in a good place so they can be calm for their child," says Dr. Rabbitts. In one study of children undergoing major surgery, she found that when parents catastrophized their children's pain prior to surgery, those children experienced higher pain intensity than a group whose parents did not. As is the case with many pain experiences, parents who are calm and collected send their children messages of confidence, and help make a difficult experience more bearable.

Even for young people who do struggle to manage pain at home after surgery, there can be a positive side to this experience:[18] "Multiple teens have told me that the skills they've learned to cope with surgery are things they're still using in their lives, and it made them a stronger or different person than they would have been," says Dr. Rabbitts. "You can use these skills to face other challenges later in life, too."

When There Is No Time to Prepare

One of Anna's most distinct childhood memories is from when she was eight years old. She was pushing closed a large sliding glass door in her family's house, and just as it was clicking shut, her two-year old sister stuck her hand into the doorframe. Through a blur of blood and screams, Anna saw that the tip of her sister's pinky finger was hanging by a thread. Anna's mom, to her credit, was able to stay calm as she told Anna to get some gauze to wrap around the finger because it was time to go to the emergency room. Anna vividly remembers sitting in the waiting room (feeling horrible) and hearing her little sister's screams as she got stitches. At the time, the screaming made sense to Anna. But now that Anna is a pediatric pain psychologist, she realizes that, even though the priority at the hospital was to reattach the fingertip, there is a lot that could have been done to ease her sister's distress. And unfortunately, in many hospitals today, the situation may not be any different.

Baruch Krauss, an associate professor of pediatrics and emergency medicine at Harvard Medical School, is working to change that. He has found that even in a fast-paced medical environment like the emergency room, where children arrive scared and in pain, physicians can build trust with them in a very short time, which is the first step in relieving their anxiety and lessening their pain.

How did he figure this out? When Dr. Krauss started working with children in the emergency room setting twenty-five years ago, he realized that he was able to calm and engage children more easily than some of his more senior colleagues. He is quick to disavow any notion that he was inherently more talented than other clinicians or had the "right personality" for dealing with children. Instead, Dr. Krauss recognized that he was using a skill set to gain children's trust, but doing so only intuitively. At that point, he couldn't quite pinpoint it. To see what was working in his own approach, he started videotaping his clinical work, and studied child development and non-verbal communication, so that he could create a methodology for what he was doing. As he puts it, he established a way "to make the intuitive obvious."

"I spent the next fifteen years deconstructing and understanding what I was doing," says Dr. Krauss, and "reconstructing it so that it's teachable to others." The core of his approach is to move children from fear to trust.[19] "It's not moving them from fear to no fear; it's moving them from fear to trust, so it's really about a relationship, about forming a human connection." Once trust is established, children are less tense and more cooperative, which can make it easier to engage them, manage their pain, and improve their overall experience with the medical procedure.

Dr. Krauss, with his blue scrubs and gentle voice, evokes the essence of Fred Rogers, minus the red sweater. His approach may be systematic but it is based in compassion, and it starts, he says, with observation. When he walks into an exam room, he takes note of the child's facial expression, behaviors, posture, and reaction to his presence. (Is the child clinging to his mother? Is he hesitant to look at you? Does he sink deeper into his mother's lap when you approach?) Dr. Krauss is also careful to observe the parent to get a sense of the emotional states that are being shared between parent and child. "There is a broadband, wireless, emotional connection between the parent and the child, and it goes both ways," he says. They feed off each other, and he's found that when he's able to connect with the child, the parent relaxes, too.

Once Dr. Krauss has interpreted the child's emotional state, he then responds with matching techniques that mirror the child's behavior. For instance, he might clasp his own hands together the way the child has clasped her hands together, all the while being mindful of physical boundaries. If the child is old enough to talk, he'll engage her in a nonthreatening way by calling her attention to an item of clothing or a physical feature that is not related to the injury. ("I see you have a pink unicorn on your shirt." "Your hair is brown and curly.") If the child seems receptive, he might move closer and ask if she wants to touch the tongue depressor in his hand. ("Do you want to hold this special tool?") All of these interactions desensitize the child to his presence and touch, capture the child's attention, and begin to build trust.

Ultimately, Dr. Krauss is able to direct the child's attention to an absorbing task, like coloring a picture, while he attends to the injury with minimal upset and pain for the child. "You use whatever methods seem to be appropriate for that particular child, and anchor their attention," he says. Fittingly, Dr. Krauss was mentored by T. Berry Brazelton, the esteemed pediatrician who transformed our modern understanding of child development. Granted, the approach Dr. Krauss uses doesn't ensure that a child will never experience any

Tips If Your Child Needs Surgery

Before the surgery:

· Consider your child's age and personality when deciding when to tell him about the surgery or procedure, and how much information to discuss. A children's book on medical visits may be a good starting point. If your child is five years or older, ask him if he has questions about what's going to happen. Answer with age-appropriate explanations.

· Ask the hospital if it offers a video or in-person tour to prepare kids for what to expect during surgery. Also find out if your child will have the help of a child life specialist at the hospital.

· Don't hesitate to call the hospital to discuss any questions or concerns you have, particularly if your child has had chronic pain or a negative experience with anesthesia. The staff should be able to go over the strategies the medical team may use to reduce the risk of persistent post-surgical pain.

· Help your child practice calming techniques, such as deep breathing, muscle relaxation, and guided imagery, in the weeks before the surgery.

· Make sure your child gets plenty of sleep in the week leading up to the surgery.

· Come prepared with distracting activities for your child to do while waiting for the procedure to begin. This is not the time to restrict screens. If there is a new app or game that your child has been wanting to try, consider saving it until the day of the surgery so he will have a novel distraction to hold his interest.

· Guide your child through relaxation techniques in the preoperative room.

After the surgery:

· Ask your child's medical team what to expect during recovery, what physical restrictions your child may have, and when he can return to regular activities. The sooner your child can get up and move around safely (without overdoing it), the better.

- Don't rely solely on opioids to manage postoperative pain. Ask your child's doctor or nurse about incorporating round-the-clock acetaminophen to minimize reliance on opioids.

- Let your child watch his favorite TV shows and video chat with friends and family; these distractions will help minimize pain and anxiety during the recovery period.

- Be aware that your child will likely need extra sleep to help his body to heal.

- Encourage your child to get back to activities gradually. If physical or occupational therapy is part of your child's postoperative care, these therapists can give guidance on how to do so.

- Seek out help if you feel that your child is highly distressed or has been traumatized by some aspect of the procedure. Children can experience trauma as a result of medical experiences, and there are specialists, including psychologists, who can help. The National Child Traumatic Stress Network also offers tip sheets to help children cope with time in the hospital and afterward. https://www.nctsn.org/what-is-child-trauma/trauma-types/medical-trauma

stress during a medical procedure. But he points out that he's less concerned about a child being a little bit stressed or uncomfortable at a certain point in the procedure than he is focused on creating a generally positive experience in the medical setting that doesn't imprint an "emotionally traumatic memory" in the child. Similar to Dr. Noel's take on memory, Dr. Krauss believes that the memories children take away from their medical experiences can have lasting consequences, but they are not immutable. "The silver lining is that a child could have ten negative experiences," he says, "and if on the eleventh experience you give them a positive experience, that almost reaches back and transforms [the negative experiences]."

Preparing for circumcision, blood draws, and other small medical procedures

Research shows that minimizing the pain of needle pricks and other minor procedures can not only make children feel more comfortable in the moment, it can also impact how much pain they feel during subsequent procedures. To prevent and alleviate discomfort, implement these strategies:

· Ask for a topical anesthetic in advance. For instance, prior to circumcision, whether it's being done by a physician or by a mohel, make sure the person performing the procedure applies a numbing cream well before making an incision.

· Provide skin-to-skin contact. Holding your baby or cuddling your older child during a procedure, such as a blood draw, can reduce stress and pain. Even holding hands can add comfort.

· Be prepared with a sweet solution. For babies, you may want to breastfeed during the procedure, or give a sugar solution, which has been shown to lessen pain. For older children, a lollipop can do the trick. If you're not able to be there, ask the person doing the procedure to give the sweet solution to your child. (There's a practical reason it's long been tradition to give babies a sweet-tasting wine-soaked cloth during religious circumcision ceremonies: it can act as a pain reliever.)

· Breathe. Remind your child to take deep breaths. For little kids, you may want to ask them to imagine they are blowing out a candle or blowing up a balloon. This naturally lowers the stress response, which in turn can lessen pain during medical procedures such as IV insertions.

· Don't focus on the procedure. Depending on your child's age, you can lessen the pain by distracting your child with a video or a conversation about the scene out the window.

· Advocate for these methods in advance. If you get pushback from a provider, remember that it's typically feasible and appropriate to provide these evidence-based, inexpensive, and pain-relieving tools to your child.

Though Dr. Krauss's method is more akin to techniques used by skilled psychologists, he has demonstrated that his method can be readily learned, and he firmly believes that it should be part of standard practice throughout healthcare. "My goal is culture change in the hospital, because you do not have to be an MD or an RN in order to read cues and respond appropriately to a child. The receptionist could do that, the X-ray tech could do that. Imagine if everyone was tuned in [to the child] in the hospital at every stage," he says. "That would be very powerful."

Chapter 6

My Tummy Hurts

*The reasons and the relief for a classic
childhood complaint*

Nolan, an athletic boy, first came into Anna's office for pain psychology counseling when he was twelve years old. He was a little shy at first, but soon began comfortably talking about his love of sports, especially football and rugby. His mom, Denise, explained that Nolan's abdominal pain had started about one year earlier when he was eleven years old, after he had been sick for a few days, throwing up. Because stomachaches are not uncommon, Denise's first thought had been that Nolan must have eaten something that didn't sit well with him or that he had gotten a virus. On one of the days, his stomach hurt so much that he couldn't get out of bed. But after the vomiting episodes stopped, he started feeling better and returned to school.

Over the next week, however, when Nolan came home from school he complained that his stomach hurt. The pain would usually feel like a deep ache around his belly button, but it sometimes turned into sharp stabs that wouldn't subside. One day, Denise remembers, it was so bad that Nolan called to be picked up early.

Denise became alarmed at that point and took Nolan to see the pediatrician that afternoon.

The doctor didn't seem too worried. She examined Nolan and asked about his pain and recent bowel movements. Because his bowel movements had become infrequent, she suggested he try a gentle laxative and add fiber to his diet to lessen constipation. Nolan's pediatrician also said that it was okay for Denise to send him to school if he didn't have a fever and was not vomiting or having diarrhea. So that's what Denise did. She made sure that Nolan ate more fruits and vegetables and sent him back to school.

It didn't take long for Denise to second-guess this advice. Nolan started going to the school nurse complaining of belly pain—and asking to go home early—at least three times a week. He also began bending over and holding his stomach after eating dinner some nights, and occasionally vomiting small amounts. Nolan's mom took him back to his pediatrician, who ran some basic tests (all were normal) and concluded this time that the discomfort might be due to acid reflux, so she prescribed a daily medication to treat that.

The medicine seemed to help alleviate the vomiting, but after a few weeks, his pain had still not subsided. What's more, Nolan had started to dread eating because it usually led to pain. Denise eliminated dairy from Nolan's diet and made sure he had plenty of fiber, but it wasn't helping. Over the next month, Nolan's pain occurred at least once every day, and when that happened, he would refuse to eat and it became hard for him to calm down. He was also feeling increasing stress about missing school and sports practices. Denise was frustrated and worried that something might be seriously wrong, so she took Nolan to the pediatrician for a third time. On this visit, the doctor did seem concerned that Nolan's pain had gone on for so long, so she referred him to a pediatric gastroenterologist at Doernbecher Children's Hospital in Portland, Oregon, where Anna works. After nearly three months of suffering, the family finally started to get some answers.

The Mysteries of Functional Gastrointestinal Disorders

While mild, short-lived tummy aches are extremely common (and we will discuss those run-of-the-mill kinds later), it turns out that Nolan is among the one in ten children in the United States with a functional gastrointestinal disorder, or FGID. This medical term can be somewhat misleading to parents because, in these cases, the stomach and intestines are not actually functioning well at all. The term simply means that, while *something* is not working properly, there is nothing structurally or biochemically wrong with the organs in the gastrointestinal tract. "The metaphor we use for functional disorders is that these are software problems rather than hardware problems," says Neil Schechter, director of the chronic pain clinic at Boston Children's Hospital.

Abdominal pain is a primary symptom of most functional gastrointestinal (GI) disorders, and many kids who suffer from recurring abdominal pain don't have any other digestive problems, such as diarrhea or acid reflux. A recent meta-analysis on FGID (distilling findings from multiple studies that were previously published) revealed that an estimated 13.5 percent of children and teens experience this type of tummy pain over and over again.[1]

Not knowing what's wrong can be incredibly difficult for families. And frustratingly, in at least 90 percent of diagnosed FGID cases, no specific medical problem with the child's digestive system is ever identified.[2] "Functional symptoms are real symptoms," says Lynn

Walker, a pediatric psychologist at Vanderbilt University Medical Center, "but the children typically show no signs of a physical disease. So these kids go to the doctor and their stomach hurts, but results of their medical evaluation are normal."

Dr. Walker has been studying functional abdominal pain, a common feature of FGID, in children for her entire research career. For one of her in-depth studies, a pediatric gastroenterology team performed thorough evaluations of 114 kids with functional abdominal pain, and found that for 107 of them (94 percent) there was no identifiable medical source for their pain.[3]

This lack of medical proof—and the fact that most physicians are not particularly familiar with treating functional abdominal pain—usually leaves children and families feeling thoroughly misunderstood. Parents frequently tell Anna that physicians they have consulted don't seem to regard their child's pain as valid. This lack of belief can cause families to doubt themselves, too.

Learning from Our Past

For most of the twentieth century, physicians were fairly obsessed with figuring out what was structurally and physiologically wrong with children who had abdominal pain. From the 1930s through the 1950s, many physicians dealt with pediatric abdominal pain by performing major exploratory surgery to investigate what was causing the problem. The doctors doing this work published case studies about their findings.[4] While some cases revealed serious abdominal problems in the children, in many cases the doctors found very minor internal redness or inflammation, or no visible problem at all, offering them minimal explanation for the pain the patients were experiencing. Cases like these suggested that surgery was not always necessary. But without X-rays, MRIs, or any other modern imaging capabilities, the doctors had no other option.

In 1958, physicians John Apley and Nora Naish conducted the first large-scale survey of abdominal pain in school-aged children in the United Kingdom.[5] Many studies have since expanded on this initial study of one thousand children, but most of their findings have stood the test of time. Dr. Apley and Dr. Naish found that, as is the case with many pain problems, girls were more likely to have belly pain than boys (12 percent versus 9 percent in their study). They identified two developmental periods in which children are particularly prone to abdominal pain: from age five to age nine, when incidence rises in both girls and boys, and from age fourteen to age fifteen, when only girls show a marked increase. They also discovered three correlations: kids with tummy pain are more likely to come from homes where there is a family history of abdominal pain, more likely to experience migraines, and more prone to anxiety and sleep problems. Well over fifty years have passed since this study was published, yet our basic understanding of the characteristics of pediatric abdominal pain has not changed. The condition still affects one in ten kids, and those kids still tend to have higher rates of anxiety and sleep problems.

Throughout the 1950s and 1960s, researchers blamed either "faulty eating habits" or "psychogenic pain" (meaning pain attributed to psychological factors) for most children's abdominal issues—mild or severe. This led pediatricians in the 1960s to draw a clear distinction between abdominal pain with "organic" (meaning physiological) versus "psychological" origins.[6] For the next decade or two, physicians and scientists espoused the belief that if they could not find anything that was physiologically wrong, it must be a psychological problem.

One notable objection to this theory came in 1967 from a pediatric surgeon named Donald G. Marshall. "To make a diagnosis of psychogenic pain, there must be something more than the absence of demonstrable organic disease," he wrote. "There must be significant psychopathology." In other words, without some evidence of a psychological condition unrelated to abdominal pain it is not valid to conclude that a child's pain has psychological origins. Dr. Marshall also noted that it is possible to have both a psychological condition *and* a separate abdominal condition. A child with a mental health condition, he pointed out, "can have appendicitis" as well. Just because there is significant psychopathology doesn't mean the source of specific pain must be psychogenic.

Dr. Marshall counseled other physicians that, in cases where there was no direct evidence for either physiological or psychological causes, they should "decide to be undecided."[7] The problem with that conclusion, however, is that human beings aren't typically comfortable with ambiguity. For most people, it feels better to get a definitive answer—either a) *the body* or b) *the mind*—than to live with uncertainty. But a definitive answer isn't always available—and scientific research in recent years on abdominal pain and how it becomes chronic has only highlighted the complexity of the human organism. The workings of our guts and brains are intertwined in intricate immune, inflammatory, and stress-response pathways. A distinction between physiological causes and psychological causes—especially with functional abdominal pain—is largely impossible.

Many people still hold the underlying conviction that there is a fundamental split between the mind and the body, despite what research reveals to the contrary. One could argue that this model of mind-body dualism has some utility in other areas of science and philosophy, but in the case of abdominal pain, this belief just does not hold up. If anything, conceptualizing the mind and body as separate has likely slowed scientific discovery into how abdominal pain really works.

Putting the Puzzle Pieces Together

Fortunately, due to public health efforts and the realization that abdominal pain is widespread (and costly), researchers have been able to study functional abdominal pain (in addition to other conditions) in larger samples of children. In the past twenty years, the expanded use of electronic medical records and other health databases has helped researchers learn much more. For instance, there are well-documented seasonal variations in rates of pediatric abdominal pain. Kids are more likely to experience this type of pain in the winter months, and less likely to experience it in the summer. Interestingly, this pattern does not show up in adult populations.[8] Instead, studies show that adults have the same rates of medical visits due to abdominal pain year-round, suggesting that there may be different underlying processes that create abdominal pain for children versus adults. Further, seasonal differences may be more pronounced in northern cities; this was the finding of a study in which researchers compared three northern cities (Wilmington, Chicago, and Pittsburgh) to three cities in Florida. All of this has led researchers to consider how a range of factors—climate, winter stomach viruses, physical activity, time spent outside, seasonal stress, circadian rhythms, daylight, and melatonin—can influence pediatric abdominal pain.[9]

In many cases, these factors come together like pieces of a puzzle to create a clearer image of how abdominal pain evolves in children.

Let's start with physical activity and time spent outdoors. Researchers suspect that, for children, engaging in these two activities is instrumental in reducing the life and school stress that kids typically experience. For children in northern cities, these vital sources of stress relief are much less available during the winter months when school-related anxiety and viral illnesses happen to be at a peak. This is unfortunate because, not only does stress increase a child's susceptibility to getting a virus, stress also increases the likelihood that children will develop persistent pain even after they've recovered from a temporary illness. Colder weather during a high-stress school period often translates to less time outside for kids to run around and blow off steam, and subsequently more chance of developing an infection and ongoing pain.

There are other puzzle pieces to consider, too, such as circadian rhythms and daylight hours. To understand how these affect abdominal pain in children, it's important to discuss melatonin, a hormone that is highly concentrated in the gut.[10] Melatonin contributes to many functions in the body, including regulation of digestion, the immune system, inflammation, and stress. The body is triggered to produce melatonin at night when we are exposed to darkness, and to suppress melatonin in the morning when we are exposed to daylight. In this way, melatonin operates as a key component in our circadian rhythms (our sleep-wake cycle, or body clock). But when day and night cycles are altered due to the short days that are characteristic of winter months in the north, melatonin production can be disrupted. And because this process is tied to the functioning of the gut, immune system, and stress, irregular melatonin production can increase a child's risk for developing abdominal pain.

Compounding matters, a child's decreased exposure to daylight during winter months in northern areas is linked with low levels of vitamin D. The power of this nutrient to affect abdominal health was shown in a recent clinical trial involving adults with irritable bowel syndrome (abdominal pain with gastrointestinal dysfunction). It demonstrated that taking vitamin D can significantly relieve people's abdominal pain and gastrointestinal symptoms, and improve quality of life.[11]

For Anna, therefore, it was notable that Nolan's abdominal pain began in early March. While it's possible that the time of year was irrelevant and his pain could just as easily have developed in any season, there is reason to suspect that factors associated with winter—circulating viruses, school stress, not nearly enough outdoor play, limited daylight, disrupted melatonin, and low levels of vitamin D—played a role. Indeed, all of these variables might have combined to set off chronic abdominal pain. Understanding a patient's condition is often a matter of fitting together different pieces of the puzzle.

How Short-Term Pain Becomes a Long-Term Problem

What few people realize is that the things that initially set off abdominal pain are often quite different from the things that keep it going. A growing body of research shows that acute illnesses like viruses and bacterial infections can lead, in children and adults, to later problems with abdominal pain and FGIDs (including irritable bowel syndrome). In some cases, the pain does not let up even years after an initial infection has resolved.[12] Among children who have had an episode of diarrhea and tested positive for infections such as rotavirus and salmonella, rates of long-lasting FGIDs and abdominal pain are about three times higher than rates seen in children who have not had an infection along with their stomach problems. In one large study involving children with confirmed gastrointestinal infections, 50 percent of the kids had persistent abdominal pain in the six-month period after the infection had resolved.[13] To be clear, not all recurrent stomach pain starts with a serious virus or infection, but the scenario is common.

How do short-term intestinal infections cause such long-term problems? One possible answer involves a complicated and developing area of study called the gut-brain axis. This term refers to the nerve signaling that goes on between the gut and the brain via the nervous system, and it can influence immune function, mood, and pain.[14] Researchers are finding that the bacterial ecosystem in the intestinal tract, called the microbiome, can set off the vagus nerve—which is the main line of communication between the gut and the brain—and affect the neuro-messages that the gut and brain send back and forth. When the bacteria in the gut are altered by an infection (which introduces pathogenic bacteria into the microbiome) or by antibiotics (which kill off both good and bad bacteria in the microbiome, upsetting typical balances), the entire gut-brain axis may begin to send mixed signals that can cause someone to feel pain, even long after the pain-causing infection is gone. Alterations in the gut-brain axis and the microbiome are also seen in anxiety, which often co-occurs with abdominal pain. Although much of this research has been done in animals, scientists think this logic applies to people, too.

Scientists are also investigating another way that short-term pain can evolve into long-term pain, having to do with a concept called visceral hyperalgesia. The term refers to a complex process whereby the viscera—the internal organs of the body, such as the stomach, liver, and intestines—become hypersensitive, likely due to changes in the gut-brain axis. The nerves in and around the intestinal tract that send messages about painful stimuli to the brain start firing more frequently than they should, causing areas in the spinal cord and brain to become more alert and responsive to pain signals. What ends up happening is that normal processes in the gut, like food moving through an intestine, set off an unnecessary alarm that the brain interprets as pain. A simpler way to explain this is to say that when kids have functional abdominal pain, their nervous system is out of whack. Visceral hyperalgesia also helps explain why, in many cases, even when the original infection that triggered the pain has resolved, the nervous system continues to behave as though the illness were still active.

Most of what we know about visceral hyperalgesia comes from studies done with animals and human adults, but the research confirms that stress can play a major role in triggering a hypersensitive gut. Animals who are exposed to infections while they are stressed are much more likely to experience persistent firing of pain signals.[15] This suggests that, if we contract an illness during a time of ongoing stress, the stress not only heightens our perception of pain signals— it can actually increase the amount of pain signaling that is coming from the nerves in our abdomen to our brain.

Researchers are also learning more about functional abdominal pain that is specific to children by studying how kids with the condition respond to mildly painful experiences in a controlled setting. For instance, Dr. Walker and her colleagues have found evidence that when kids with functional abdominal pain are exposed to painful stimuli elsewhere on their body, their pain modulation systems don't seem to work at an optimal level, causing them to have a heightened sensitivity to that new source of pain.[16]

Other studies of children with functional abdominal pain have employed a test called the cold pressor task (CPT) to show how stress impacts pain tolerance. In the CPT, children are instructed to keep their hand in a tub of very cold water until it becomes too painful. This simple measure of pain tolerance has given researchers significant insight into factors that influence pain responses in children. In one study involving kids with abdominal pain, researchers had half of the children undergo a relatively basic stressor (the children were interviewed about stress and had to complete a difficult math problem out loud) prior to doing the CPT. The other half of the children with abdominal pain did the CPT first. The results were illuminating. The kids who underwent the stressor first had much lower pain tolerance compared to the kids who did the CPT first. In other words, exposure to stress directly influenced the children's pain tolerance in the moment.[17]

All told, this research tells us that, in Nolan's case, and for many children like him, a cascade of neurophysiologic changes can lead to pain and hypersensitivity. It's highly plausible that Nolan had a virus that set off inflammation and pain in his stomach. But even after his body successfully fought off the virus, winter school stress coupled with his limited access to outdoor play paved the way for him to develop visceral hyperalgesia (a super-sensitive gut), which amped up his pain-sensing system during normal digestive processes. Nolan's heightened discomfort then caused him to miss more school days and experience more stress, which further hindered his ability to tolerate pain. The cycle of pain and stress then continued on auto-loop, resulting in an unrelenting pattern that many abdominal pain patients don't seem to be able to break.

Helping Patients Understand

Not all physicians receive training in the neurobiological mechanisms of the gut-brain axis and visceral hyperalgesia. But imagine you are a physician who does understand how the nervous system gets sensitized in the gut and brain, and you are 99 percent sure this is what's happening in one of your patients. How do you explain this concept in everyday language to a parent, much less to a child, so that it makes sense and does not inadvertently imply their pain is all in their heads? It isn't easy. And that's part of the reason many families dealing with functional abdominal pain remain confused about what's going on.

We know, however, from the work of Sara Williams, who is one of Dr. Walker's former graduate students, that the way physicians talk about and explain functional abdominal pain really matters. Dr. Williams conducted a study involving mothers in which they were each asked to imagine that their child had abdominal pain. They rated how distressing the situation was to them and then watched one of four videos. Each video was of a pediatrician offering a different explanation for a child's abdominal pain, along with recommendations about how to alleviate it. The mothers who were told that there was no medical basis for their child's pain were more distressed and less satisfied than the mothers who were told that the child had functional abdominal pain—and were given an explanation of what that means and how stress management can alleviate the symptoms.[18] Paradoxically, while there are physicians who are trained in diagnosing functional abdominal pain, they are not always well-equipped to explain functional disorders in a way that families are likely to understand.

Communication between practitioners and patients can also be strained when there are racial and cultural differences—or language barriers—between them. Andrew Campbell, director of the sickle cell program at Children's National Hospital in Washington, DC, says that it can be hard for providers and patients to relate to each other and understand each other when they don't have shared cultural experiences between them. "Some of it has to do with the providers' implicit racial bias that we see, and some of it has to do with patients' learned distrust of medicine," he says.[19] But he notes that when there *is* a racial or cultural connection, this can open up the lines of communication and improve trust between providers and patients. "Sometimes just being an African American physician walking into the exam room to a family of color, I can see their guards come down. They're more receptive, and feel they can speak more openly about things and won't be judged," says Dr. Campbell, who is also an associate professor of pediatrics at George Washington University School of Medicine and Health Sciences. "I can also talk about things that other physicians may not be able to or may feel uncomfortable talking about."

For healthcare practitioners who don't share the same racial or cultural background as their patients, Dr. Campbell says there are still ways they can connect with each other. "The first step is listening to your patients and believing them," he says. Another critical strategy is to give families time to absorb information and treatment recommendations. "I recognize that some families need to have the opportunity to digest something new. So I like to present the information and say what I recommend, and say we can talk about it at the next visit because I understand having questions, and I know families are much more likely to go to their appointments and follow treatment recommendations if they feel their provider listens to them and cares about them."

Helping Doctors Understand the Patient

There is another plausible—and surprisingly simple—reason it took Nolan's pediatrician so long to recognize his abdominal pain as a serious problem: tummy pain is one of the most common reasons that kids go to the doctor. What's more, physicians don't worry much about these cases because abdominal pain is a single symptom and most often is not a sign of a life-threatening illness. If a child doesn't have a fever or intestinal blockage, and does not show other signs of serious illness, physicians may not even order an X-ray because, statistically speaking, nothing is likely to be wrong (plus, radiation exposure should be avoided unless it's necessary). And, perhaps most importantly, physicians see many pediatric patients with abdominal pain get better over time with minimal treatment.

By contrast, when parents see their child in pain, they often observe a dramatic shift in the child's general demeanor. Nolan's mom described how he changed from being a really active boy who played sports and loved spending time with his teammates to being a child who would often be curled up in bed, unable to do much of anything other than distract himself with video games. Parents see what physicians can't glimpse in the exam room: a child sobbing uncontrollably in the middle of the night; a child who no longer talks about friends or asks to see them; a child who has to be coaxed to get out of bed in the morning. When parents are living this day in and day out, it is hard for them to imagine that anything except a serious illness could cause such a severe change in their child.

In Nolan's case, even after his pediatrician finally referred him to a gastroenterologist, it took two more months before the specialist was able to see Nolan for an appointment. (Wait times are often up to six months for pediatric specialty care in the United States.) These long wait times often breed more worry for families. Many parents tell Anna that watching their child go through serious pain day after day makes it hard not to think about the worst possible outcomes.

As we now know, the longer children worry and wait for their pain to be addressed, the more their nervous systems change in response to that pain and stress. And this maladaptive learning—which in the case of abdominal pain can cause long-lasting alterations to the gut-brain axis—makes it much more likely that a child's pain will become chronic and disabling. The lesson, then, is simple: the sooner we help kids cope with pain, the more likely they are to recover.

The Link between Stomach Pain and Mood Disorders

In Nolan's case, he did not benefit from treatment right away. Instead, for several months, he experienced pain almost every day. As pediatric psychologists know, chronic pain can disrupt more than physical functioning, sleep patterns, and school attendance. It can also derail a child's emotional functioning and friendships.

The medical community is learning more and more about the long-term impact of pediatric abdominal pain, again thanks to Dr. Walker, this time due to her work with adults who had functional abdominal pain in childhood. Her research reveals that early abdominal pain is related to increased lifetime risk for anxiety disorders. So a bellyache that doesn't go away might be an early sign of anxiety that could continue as the child gets older. Not all kids do, but a substantial portion of kids with chronic abdominal pain experience a period of significant anxiety or depression by early adulthood. In a 2013 study that evaluated a sample of children with functional abdominal pain that had been followed through young adulthood by Dr. Walker, researchers found that about half of the people who had functional abdominal pain in childhood had an anxiety disorder in their lifetime. By comparison, of the people who didn't have childhood abdominal pain, only 12 percent had an anxiety disorder throughout their life. The pattern is similar for depression with 40 percent of people who had childhood abdominal pain experiencing depression at some point compared to only 16 percent of people who didn't have a history of an abdominal problem.[20] Tragically, this work also shows that there is also a significant portion of people who never seem to beat their abdominal pain; they go on to be diagnosed with functional gastrointestinal disorders (FGID) as adults.

Tackling Tummy Problems

There *is* an upside to this research. It shows that if we can successfully address stomachaches in children before they become a larger problem, we may be able to stem the tide of functional abdominal pain in childhood and reduce the rates of FGIDs, anxiety, and depression in adulthood.[21]

It's fair to conclude that medical providers *should* worry about kids with functional abdominal pain. In fact, we should all worry more about these kids. We should worry about the impact the pain is having on their school attendance and physical functioning, and we should recommend treatments that can support them.

It's also important to be aware that many of the cognitive-behavioral therapies (CBT) that can alleviate chronic functional abdominal pain are also effective in relieving short-term tummy troubles, no matter the cause. CBT methods have been shown in numerous studies to improve children's abilities to cope with pain, lessen its impact, and return to daily activities.[22]

Cognitive Behavioral Strategies for Treating Abdominal Pain (Short-Term or Long-Term)

If abdominal pain arises, and if it persists, there are cognitive behavioral strategies that can help.

- **Try relaxation techniques.** As we've discussed, stress can intensify pain. Deep breathing and guided imagery can lessen the sensation of pain by impacting areas of the brain that are involved in pain signaling.

- **Look for distractions.** One of the lessons we learned from Chapter 3 is that when we focus on pain, it can make it feel worse. When kids feel stomach pain, they often benefit from engaging in an absorbing activity such as reading a good book or watching a movie.
- **Practice good sleep habits.** Too little sleep can make pain more problematic. Help your child get enough sleep by establishing a regular bedtime and wake time to keep sleep consistent. Limit electronics and screen usage right before bed to encourage the production of melatonin prior to sleeping. Avoid physical activity, big meals, or caffeine shortly before bed, which can rev up the body and make it difficult to wind down for sleep. Discourage anxiety-inducing activities before bed, such as homework. Keep the bedroom cool and dark, which is conducive to sleep.
- **Participate in normal activities.** When children focus only on their pain and are removed from their everyday lives, this can lead to increased pain, isolation, anxiety, and depression. Encourage your child to take part in school, social events, and after-school activities. If pain flares, remind your child to use deep breathing, distraction, or other coping techniques rather than going home at the first sign of discomfort.
- **Avoid unhelpful thoughts.** It's common for children to develop intense fear and worry about their pain and experience thoughts such as "my pain will never go away." (This is sometimes called "catastrophizing"). But these thoughts can make the experience of pain worse. Work

with your child (or engage a therapist) to help him identify these unhelpful thoughts and shift thinking toward
more positive outcomes, such as "I can manage my pain
with deep breathing."

- **Keep the lines of communication open.** It's crucial that we
don't forget about children's psychological functioning in
the midst of pain, and that we provide screening and
treatment for any symptoms of anxiety and depression
that kids may have along with their pain.

Finding Relief

Nolan finally got on a path toward pain relief. His gastroenterologist had him undergo several additional tests, including an endos-
copy with biopsies, to be sure he did not have a serious underlying
disease. When these tests all came back normal, the gastroenterologist explained that Nolan was, in fact, experiencing real pain, and
that it was due to a problem with his nerves being overly sensitive
after an illness. The doctor made clear that Nolan's pain-signaling
system was influenced by stress and could be made better through
relaxation and other techniques. As well as prescribing a medication
that reduces muscle spasms in the bowel, the gastroenterologist recommended a few diet modifications, and suggested that, for Nolan's
pain to resolve, he might need psychosocial support to get back to
school and learn to relax his body. (Some gastroenterologists also
recommend supplementing with probiotics—good bacteria that may
help restore balance in the microbiome and improve gut health—
although studies on this show mixed results.)[23]

That's when Nolan was referred to Anna, who learned that although Denise was no longer worried about Nolan having a life-

threatening illness, she was very concerned about what would happen if he continued to have pain. He would be entering middle school in a few months, and Denise was nervous that he would fall behind academically and that middle-school teachers would not be as accommodating as his elementary teacher had been. All of this worry caused Denise to be hyper-focused on helping Nolan get better. She was jumping in to try to help him every time he had pain by encouraging him to rest after meals. She was also watching him closely to be sure that he didn't eat foods that seemed to trigger his pain, and she often suggested that he should take a break from sports.

Anna explained to Denise that this extra help—no matter how well-intentioned—was probably communicating her anxiety to Nolan and sending him the message that he might not be able to handle his pain on his own. Anna talked with Nolan and Denise about how Nolan might be able to use relaxation techniques and other biobehavioral strategies to manage his pain episodes on his own. He was particularly worried about pain after eating, and with some trial and error he found that a mindful walk or short bike ride right after dinner really helped him keep his mind off his stomachache.

After a few visits with Anna, Nolan also shared that he was worried about the pain happening at school because he didn't want to seem different from his friends or call attention to himself in this way. As with many children who've missed school because of pain, he started to feel that some of the kids at school were being mean to him or ignoring him. With some counseling from Anna and a bit of creative problem-solving, Nolan was able to reconnect with friends and worry less about what other kids might think.

Nolan also learned to be aware of when he felt stress in his body, and then used the deep breathing techniques Anna had taught him to relax, which ultimately lessened the severity of his pain episodes. Slowly but surely, both Nolan and Denise became more confident in Nolan's ability to manage the pain. The last Anna heard from Denise, Nolan was going to rugby practice, was rarely missing school, and was continuing to work with his pediatrician and gastroenterologist. With the tools he needed, Nolan was getting back to the business of being an active young boy.

Chapter 7

When the Pain *Is* in Your Head

Management of frequent headaches—
which should never be ignored

The migraines started when Mina was thirteen years old. About once a month, she would feel a sudden throbbing pressure encircling the front of her head like an unyielding metal headband. There were no warning signs—no blurred vision or floating bright dots, which can precede migraines. Instead, she would be hit with jarring discomfort, seemingly out of nowhere.

"It would start hurting and be up to the worst part within ten minutes of the start of the migraine," says Mina, who also became nauseous, dizzy, and sensitive to light with each episode—all symptoms that often accompany migraines. "That fast onset made it so that a lot of rescue medications would not help me, because they take about fifteen minutes to work."

Rescue medications, as Mina quickly learned, are pain relievers such as acetaminophen (Tylenol), which is an analgesic, and ibuprofen (Advil or Motrin), which is a nonsteroidal anti-inflammatory drug (NSAID). Mina tried these medications because they had always helped her dad with his migraines. (Yes, migraines often run in families). But these over-the-counter (OTC) medications were not enough help for Mina, who is now twenty years old. Once a migraine set in, she could not function. Her only recourse was to lie in her bed in her darkened room, for days.

"In the beginning, the headache would last probably three days and would keep me from school," remembers Mina, who at that time lived with her parents and younger sister in Portland, Oregon. "The NSAIDs would take the pain down a little bit—and towards the end of the three days, I would be able to get out of bed and do some basic things, like some homework, but looking at a computer screen would be too much."

In eighth grade, the monthly migraines weren't "that big of a deal," says Mina. Missing three days of school each month was hard, but "doable."

But over the course of Mina's freshman and sophomore years of high school, the migraines got more intense and lasted longer. Over-the-counter medications stopped having any effect, so her pediatrician prescribed Imitrex (generic name: sumatriptan), which is a common first line of treatment for migraines. "It worked for around three months," Mina recalls, "and then it just stopped working altogether."

The pediatrician eventually referred Mina to a pediatric neurologist, who ordered an MRI. The imaging test didn't reveal any specific underlying issue so the neurologist prescribed different migraine medications. "After Imitrex, he prescribed Topamax and then Maxalt—which didn't work for me—and then he said there was nothing left for me."

The headaches got worse. By the time Mina began her junior year of high school, each migraine would last a week to two weeks, and in addition to the migraines she developed chronic daily tension headaches. There was no end to the pain, not even for one day.

Mina went to another neurologist and tried a litany of medications. Of the twenty drugs she tried over the years, some didn't work for her, some caused unbearable side effects (such as extreme fatigue, dizziness, memory loss, drop in blood pressure, lack of appetite, and weight loss), and some were both ineffective and intolerable.

And those were just the medications. Mina also tried complementary therapies, which didn't offer her much relief. First, she sought out well-known modalities, including chiropractic treatment and massage. Then she tried lesser known approaches such as transcutaneous electrical nerve stimulation (TENS), which involves placing electrode pads on or near the area of pain. During a TENS treatment, pulses are sent via the pads through the skin and along the nerve fibers in an effort to suppress pain signals to the brain and prompt the body to produce higher levels of its own pain-reducing chemicals. But this therapy had no pain-relieving effects for Mina. One nerve-stimulation device she tried, with the brand name Cephaly, sends micro-impulses to the upper branch of the trigeminal nerve through a magnetic electrode. Mina describes the pricey product this way: "It looks like a crown on your head that you wear for ten minutes a day. I was able to rent it from my neurologist's office. It was weird and it didn't help."

Mina also tried an elimination diet, giving up gluten and dairy for four months to determine if those foods were migraine triggers, but the change to eating habits proved ineffective and only made her and her parents' lives more difficult. There is research showing that eliminating certain dietary triggers—the most common being caffeine, monosodium glutamate (MSG), cocoa, aspartame, and cheese—can reduce or even eliminate headaches in children.[1] It doesn't, however, work for everyone. Plus, as Mina's family discovered, trying to adhere to a strict diet can add stress to an already stressful situation. Anna has often seen elimination diets turn into a source of family conflict because they place yet more restrictions on teens who, under typical circumstances, would increasingly be making their own decisions about what they eat. When a family does try an elimination diet, Anna also encourages working with a physician or registered dietician to make sure that the child's overall health and nutrition needs are considered.[2]

For Mina, nearing the end of eleventh grade, it felt as though she'd exhausted all of her options. Gone from her life were the after-school activities she had enjoyed, like jujitsu and dance. And with pain so frequently making it impossible for her to read, focus on a computer screen, or think critically, she fell behind in her studies. "Junior year was especially rough. I had always been a straight-A student, but my head hurt all the time and I was missing a lot of school—and most of my teachers didn't understand," remembers Mina. "I got two letters from the district saying if I missed any more school I wouldn't be able to graduate. I was stubborn and I didn't ask for help until the very last minute when I was failing all my classes and the quarter was about to end."

At that point, Mina's guidance counselor got her parents and teachers together and they were able to put in place accommodations to help her get back on track. Specifically, Mina's school developed a "504 plan" for her, so-called because it delivers on rights specified in section 504 of the Rehabilitation Act of 1973, a major piece of US federal law designed to ensure that children with health limitations or disabilities are given equal opportunities, including the tools they need to succeed in school. (For more on individualized 504 plans, see Chapter 12.) "That made it a little better," Mina says, "but I ended up having to drop three classes out of eight that semester. I'd never done that before, and that was very stressful."

On top of that, Mina didn't have much peer support. "I didn't have many friends at school, partially because I was never there," she says. "And when I was there, I didn't want to talk to anybody because I hurt really bad, or I was tired, or all of the above."

Unsurprisingly, Mina began to develop severe anxiety. Between headaches, school stress, social isolation, and lack of positive outlets, she started having panic attacks at least once a week.

It was around that time that Mina was referred to OSHU's Comprehensive Pain Center where she began seeing Anna (as her pediatric pain psychologist) as well as a pain physician and a physical therapist. Seeing a psychologist was not a new experience for Mina but this would be her first time working with a practitioner specifically trained and experienced in counseling children with chronic pain. Anna was familiar with the special circumstances of such patients, and had seen many kids like Mina before.

An All-Too-Common Condition

Given how long Mina struggled with migraines and tension headaches—and how little relief her doctors were able to offer—one would think she'd been dealing with a relatively rare condition. But headaches are one of the most common childhood disorders. More than ten million children and adolescents in the United States have recurrent headaches, according to the National Headache Foundation—and that's about 20 percent of children ages five to seventeen. Broken down into types of headaches, an estimated 15 percent of all children have recurring tension headaches, and another 5 percent have migraines. Many additional children, of course, experience occasional headaches but don't suffer regularly. Surveys indicate that 75 percent of children have had a significant headache by the age of fifteen, and over three hundred thousand children, desperate for relief, arrive at emergency departments with headaches each year.[3]

Statistics also show that as kids get older, problems with headaches become more common. One study of twelve- to seventeen-year-olds found that about 50 percent of boys and 75 percent of girls had had a headache in the past month, with fourteen- to seventeen-year-old girls experiencing the highest incidence of migraines. And tragically, there are many children, like Mina, who endure intractable migraines or chronic daily headaches that don't subside despite medication and other interventions. For these kids, pain is a constant and often debilitating part of their lives—and in most cases, their chronic headaches continue into adulthood.[4]

The good news: most pediatric headaches are benign, meaning they are not connected to a cancerous tumor or other life-threatening brain abnormality. And for many children, it doesn't take long to get an accurate diagnosis, which is the first step toward a viable treatment. "One thing about migraine patients is that they often get a diagnosis faster than other pediatric patients with more mysterious diagnoses that practitioners wouldn't know outside of a pain clinic," says Emily Law, a pediatric pain psychologist and assistant professor of pain medicine at Seattle Children's Research Institute.

The not-so-good news: Even though headache patients often know their diagnosis, it can take just as long for them to get comprehensive help (or to reach a pain clinic) as it does for children with less obvious conditions, says Dr. Law. So it is not uncommon for children with headaches to suffer for years trying to nail down an effective treatment plan.

Uncertain Causes

Chronic headaches can be particularly vexing because they are usually brought on by a culmination of many factors—such as genetics, trauma, hormonal fluctuations, infection, exposure to environmental stimuli (like certain foods or sunlight), and lifestyle habits (like sleep deprivation or dehydration). With so many factors at play, the causes and triggers of headaches can vary greatly from person to person.

In some cases, headaches are triggered by injuries or other health conditions, such as concussions, vision problems, Lyme disease, or sinus problems. In these instances, the headaches need to be evaluated as a possible symptom of a larger problem. Often, identifying potential lifestyle triggers—and managing them—can be invaluable to alleviating headaches. But for the majority of children dealing with headaches, there is no clear source, particularly if the headaches are frequent and chronic. Not being able to pinpoint a cause can be incredibly frustrating for them and their parents.

For migraines, researchers haven't identified a definitive physiological cause for their occurrence, but they have developed a theory. The theory is based on current understanding of allostasis, which is the process by which the body adapts to and copes with the many stressors that constantly threaten its homeostasis—that is, its baseline stability. Keep in mind that these stressors can be environmental (like missing the bus), psychosocial (getting bullied or worrying that someone won't like you), psychological (feeling anxious), or physical (being dehydrated, experiencing a hormonal shift, or not getting enough sleep)—and our bodies don't know the difference. Under average circumstances, when a person is confronted with a limited number of stressors, allostasis tends to work pretty well: a stressor pops up, the body reacts to it via hormonal and neural mediators, and our bodies and brains quickly return to homeostasis. At baseline, the body is ready to respond to the next stressor. But when there are multiple stressors coming at us (chronic or severe), our stress response system can get pushed beyond what it can handle and become dysregulated. In some cases, the cumulative burden—or "allostatic load"—becomes so great that the brain essentially fails to turn off the stress response, and migraines occur.[5]

Children may be able to visualize this concept by imagining that their baseline physiological state is a toy boat floating along in a bathtub, and the stressors in their lives are non-floating toys placed on board the boat—perhaps solid plastic mermaids, animals, and pirate loot. Kids who are sleep-deprived or stressed already have plenty of toys in their boat, and perhaps are struggling to stay afloat. When even more toys come on board (in the form of an external stressor like a midterm exam or an ear infection), the boat may sink, and trigger a migraine. To avoid this, kids can take stock of the toys, or stressors in their lives, and find ways to lessen the load. For some kids, there may be lots of minor stressors (like too many after-school activities) and they might be able to eliminate some of those. For others, throwing one big stressor overboard (like a chronic lack of sleep) might steady the boat.

To make matters more complicated, having migraines is a stressor in and of itself, so a vicious cycle can emerge in which seemingly minor stressors can trigger major headaches. With so many variables conspiring together to cause chronic headaches, it can take a great deal of trial and error to arrive at effective treatments and create a state of smooth sailing.

Treatment Benefits, Side Effects, and Expectations

For patients like Mina, the road to the right treatment approach (or even to an established pain program or headache clinic) can be long and winding—and filled with many detours. "By the time I see patients at a pain clinic, there's often a lot of frustration, questions, and anger," says Mark Connelly, a pediatric psychologist and co-director of the Comprehensive Headache Clinic at Children's Mercy Hospital and Clinics in Kansas City, Missouri. "And, as with other patients with chronic pain, they've sometimes gotten the message that the pain is 'in their head,' meaning it's purely psychological or not real."

Let's pause for a moment on that expression, "it's all in your head." As Dr. Connelly notes, someone using that phrase is not implying that patients actually have significant pain in their heads (which is literally the case with headaches), but rather that their pain is purely emotional, not physically real. Yet it's critical to remember that, in the case of headaches and many other forms of pain, psychological factors do affect physical symptoms. This hardly means that the pain can be dismissed as a figment of the imagination. It does mean, however, that psychological factors must be recognized and addressed. As discussed above, certain psychological stressors can make pain worse. Fortunately, as we've learned, psychological strategies can also be harnessed and implemented to alleviate pain.

For instance, landmark research led by Scott Powers, pediatric psychologist and co-director of the Headache Center at Cincinnati

Children's Medical Center, found that a placebo pill can be just as effective at treating childhood migraines as two of the most common migraine medications—topiramate (brand name: Topamax) and amitriptyline (brand name: Elavil)—and may be even more effective.

When Dr. Powers and his colleagues designed their trial, the intention was not to prove the placebo effect. There was already a body of research showing that if patients are given fake remedies, but are not aware of that and believe the medications will work, they can experience neurobiological healing effects that are surprisingly powerful.[6] Instead, this study's use of placebo pills was merely to provide a control group in a large, randomized, double-blind, placebo-controlled trial evaluating the effects of two migraine medications in children ranging in age from eight to seventeen. In such trials, patients are randomly assigned to receive either a placebo pill or a medication, and neither the patients nor the clinicians know who is receiving which; both sides are "blind" to this information until after the study is completed.[7]

"To our surprise, at the first interim analysis, while not statistically different, the placebo group was doing better than the two drug groups, and the two drug groups were doing about the same—with a reduction of 50 percent or more in headache frequency," says Dr. Powers. "So we stopped the trial. The drugs didn't meet the standard of efficacy that we thought they would and, at the conclusion of the trial, if you just took it on straight data, the medicines weren't more effective than placebo—and they had more side effects. Therefore, the risk-benefit of prescribing the medicines was, at best, suspect." This study does not suggest that drugs are never effective for childhood migraines, or that the placebo effect was a fluke. On the contrary, as Dr. Powers says, "the number one 'take home' of the study was that 50 to 65 percent of the time, kids with migraines get better."

The research highlights that there are various ways to get better. If you look at the headache literature in general, Dr. Connelly notes, "somewhere between 50 to 65 percent of kids with headaches are going to improve no matter what the treatment is." Why, then, do some kids get better with medication, some improve even with a placebo, and some benefit from another approach? "The positive outcome probably has something to do with your belief in the treatment already," Dr. Connelly says. "So if you line up your beliefs with your treatment, you'll have a better chance of success." In other words, he says, "Maybe the underlying mechanism is that it's not the treatment per se, but the expectation that something will work. We have a fair amount of treatments, ranging from cognitive behavioral therapy and medication to acupuncture or a combination of modalities. So with an interdisciplinary model, if we can match up the patient's perception of what's going to be beneficial, it can maximize expectancy or the placebo effect."[8]

Some research shows that when people expect a treatment to work, even if they are told it's a placebo or a sugar pill, it can trigger actual neurochemical changes and alleviate pain. Ted J. Kaptchuk, a professor of medicine at Harvard Medical School, has spent much of his career conducting studies on the placebo effect, and his work has illustrated that the ritual of being given medicine by a trusted authority (even if that medicine consists of a sugar pill) can make people feel significantly better. Mindset matters.[9]

As the latest headache research causes scientists and clinicians to reconsider why kids with headaches get better, cognitive behavioral therapy (CBT) has gained supporters. As Dr. Powers says, "CBT has achieved fairly comparable effects to medication, and we're seeing more psychologists treating pain than we've had before." Still, he cautions, there is "that 20 percent to 30 percent of kids with

Headache Basics

Determining the best treatments for your child's headaches can take trial and error. These general guidelines can help you get started.

- See your pediatrician for an evaluation if your child is experiencing headaches more than two times per week.

- Limit over-the-counter pain medications to no more than twice a week; in some people, overuse of medication causes rebound headaches. Also, heavy long-term use of analgesics can cause damage to the stomach, liver, and kidneys.

- Be mindful of lifestyle factors, which affect headaches (including migraines) more than most people realize. When children struggle with headaches, the easiest first steps are for them to get adequate sleep, stay hydrated, and engage in moderate amounts of physical activity most days.

- Promote self-efficacy by encouraging children to take charge of their well-being—for example by drinking more water or getting more sleep—especially as they enter adolescence. If your teenager is reluctant, consider working with a psychologist or behavioral medicine consultant.

If headaches follow a concussion—defined as a blow to the head that can cause damage to brain cells—more specific guidance applies. (Concussion is also discussed briefly in Chapter 8.) This is a type of traumatic brain injury and is typically considered mild if a person does not lose consciousness from the blow, or if the person was unconscious for less than thirty minutes after impact. But even mild concussions need to be taken seriously.* To increase the chances of a speedy recovery, make use of these strategies:

- Consult a healthcare provider as soon as possible after a concussion to assess the degree of injury.

- Encourage your child to rest, nap, and get plenty of sleep after a concussion, especially in the first few days of recovery. Common symptoms of concussion—headaches, poor concentration, irritability, fatigue, and memory problems—often dissipate with adequate rest and sleep.

- Take it slowly as your child returns to activities after a concussion. Doing too much too soon can trigger symptoms. Studies have shown that when people are given instructions on how to gradually return to activities after a concussion, the length of time they experience symptoms can be reduced.[†]

- Tell your child to expect improvements within a week of a concussion, and anticipate that headaches will gradually fade. Research shows that positive expectations may actually help recovery.[‡]

- Consider relaxation, guided imagery, or other bio-behavioral techniques for managing pain, in addition to any medications that your child's healthcare provider prescribes.

- See your healthcare provider if your child is still experiencing headaches a month after a concussion. The vast majority of children who experience concussions make a full recovery within one week to a month.

---

[*] W. Mittenberg, R. Zielinski, and S. Fichera, "Recovery from Mild Head Injury: A Treatment Manual for Patients," *Psychotherapy in Private Practice* 12, no. 2 (1993): 37–52; R. L. Zemek, K. J. Farion, M. Sampson, and C. McGahern, "Prognosticators of Persistent Symptoms Following Pediatric Concussion: A Systematic Review," *JAMA Pediatrics* 167, no. 3 (2013): 259–265.

[†] W. Mittenberg, G. Tremont, R. E. Zielinski, S. Fichera, and K. R. Rayls, "Cognitive-Behavioral Prevention of Postconcussion Syndrome," *Archives of Clinical Neuropsychology* 11, no. 2 (1996): 139–145.

[‡] W. Mittenberg, D. V. DiGiulio, S. Perrin, and A. E. Bass, "Symptoms Following Mild Head Injury: Expectation as Aetiology," *Journal of Neurology, Neurosurgery and Psychiatry* 55, no. 3 (1992): 200–204.

[persistent] migraines and we probably have to work a little harder to figure out what's going to be helpful to them. Because this is a real disease. It's certainly not just in their head."

Dr. Powers is also determined to figure out how to prevent children with migraines from becoming adults with migraines. "What happens to a forty-five-year-old woman that has migraines—whose brain has been impacted by pain for twenty-five years? Is that brain functioning differently in pain processing? I certainly have a belief that the developing brain is where we want to get migraine under control."

Managing Migraines

Despite the prevalence of migraines in children, Dr. Law at Seattle Children's reports hearing regularly from people that they didn't know kids could even get migraines. Yet she has spent the bulk of her career researching and treating children in pain—with a focus on headaches. "If there is one thing I want to make clear," she says, "it's that kids get migraines, too—and they're just as disabling as they are for adults."

But there is hope, as Mina can attest. Her headaches finally began to improve after she found the pain clinic at OHSU and started working with her current pain physician, Kimberly Mauer, and with Anna. Granted, there was (and still is) a fair bit of trial and error involved in her treatment. "Going into my senior year of high school, my doctor and I started trying trigger point injections, a phenoganglion drip, and an occipital nerve block—all of which involve needles or sticking something up your nose and they didn't work, which was frustrating," remembers Mina. But at the pain clinic, Mina finally felt that her doctors were on her side and would not give up on finding an effective treatment plan for her.

Also, Anna taught Mina how to cope with her headaches a bit more effectively. "She helped me realize that this was probably going to continue for a while and I couldn't just stop living my life." Cognitive behavioral tools and strategies helped to minimize the pain and its impact on her activities. A turning point for Mina was when she learned to view her headache pain as an inconvenience rather than an emergency. Why was this so important? Research shows that having negative thoughts about pain—fears like "this is only going to get worse" or "I'll never be able to handle college"—can increase the intensity of pain we experience. When kids practice the skill of thinking more positively, it can help them focus on what they want to do with their lives, rather than on what pain is keeping them from doing.

Mina also began to notice that when she did less because of headaches, her mood started to deteriorate, but when she participated in things that were important to her (like going to school and spending time with friends), she felt happier—and that mood improvement enabled her to cope better when she had more intense headaches. With Anna's help, Mina assessed which activities she wanted to be sure to participate in, and together they problem-solved ways to be engaged in these valued activities as much as possible despite her pain. Together, they figured out what worked best for Mina in terms of boosting her spirits, lowering her anxiety, and reducing her pain.

Over the course of Mina's senior year she gained the ability to manage school even with migraines. Although she still didn't feel great every day, she gradually found ways to cope. For example, because lack of sleep would exacerbate Mina's headaches, she arranged her schedule so that she didn't have early-morning classes, which gave her time to get more sleep. Mina also became proactive about asking her teachers for breaks during the day, which gave her eyes time to rest and enabled her to get through classes with less pain than the previous year. She also started doing deep breathing exercises that Anna taught her. "They helped me calm down and refocus," says Mina, who ended up missing far fewer days of school during her senior year. Additionally, instead of spending valuable energy trying to identify a single stressor that needed to be erased in order to fix her headaches, Mina started thinking about the larger group of stressors that her body and brain might be experiencing. This enabled her to view lifestyle factors—like getting more sleep and staying hydrated—as part of an overall stress reduction plan, which helped her feel more in control of her migraine treatment.

One of the biggest shifts for Mina was her mindset. "It was an attitude change. Dr. Wilson told me that pain is like your fight-or-flight response—sort of like your brain freaking out because you think something is wrong. But for me, with my headaches, nothing is actually wrong with my brain. It's just how I'm feeling at the moment, so that doesn't mean that I have to stop what I'm doing when I have a headache."

Indeed, though humans are conditioned to stop what we're doing when we experience pain (as discussed in Chapter 1, it's our body's protective response to pull our hand away from a hot burner as soon as we touch it and feel the burn), not all pain is a valid warning signal that actions must be halted. And if we can find a way to move through unnecessary pain, we can help train our nervous system to relegate that pain to the sidelines.

It's important to note that Mina's new attitude was not based on the premise that she should dismiss her pain as though it weren't real. Rather, her new attitude was based on the idea that she would be okay, and she could still participate in life, even with pain. This framework is crucial for managing chronic pain, and it is most effective when patients are supported in this belief by their family and clinicians.

"When we started the Headache Center at Cincinnati Children's in 1996, our first foundational block was that we would never see a patient or a family that doesn't know we believe them and that they have a whole team behind them," says Dr. Powers. His reasoning was that his patients' success depends on this shared understanding.

Dr. Law echoes this sentiment and explains that a big part of her role as a pediatric pain psychologist is to validate her patients' experience. "I have lots of kids with migraines who have been to provider after provider and they tell me that they've been told they made up their pain—and that's so unhelpful," says Dr. Law. "So we'll say things like 'Your pain is real and you've got a team of people who really care about you and we're here for you, and we're going to help you feel better.'"[10]

Mina is now in college. She's feeling challenged and excited by her classes, is getting good grades, and is having fun spending time with friends. She found a neurologist near her and started going to yoga classes with a friend to help her continue her relaxation practice. In other words, she has learned to live on her own and stay involved in things that are meaningful to her—even when she's battling migraines. Importantly, Mina emerged from an extremely stressful time in high school with a strong sense of independence and self-efficacy around managing her pain. She is also optimistic about her future—hoping to become a physical therapist. No doubt, her own experiences with pain, multidisciplinary therapies, and perseverance will help her excel in guiding others to manage pain, to heal, and to live fully.

Chapter 8

Too Much Pain, No Gain

*The rise of sports injuries—and how
to avoid sidelining young athletes*

Hannah exuded strength and confidence as she ran through the wooded trails of Amherst, Massachusetts. The high-school senior with a small, five-foot-one frame and lean muscles loved running and was a top athlete on her school's cross-country and track teams. She especially relished cross-country season, which she'd participated in every fall since freshman year. She'd spend hour after meditative hour traversing leafy paths, breathing in fresh air, and feeling the rhythm of her cadence through every sinewy fiber of her body.

Hannah also thrived on setting goals and achieving them. "I trained hard and saw results," she says. More training led to better running times. "It was very concrete, and I found it very empowering." She felt a kinship with her teammates who also valued discipline, cheered each other on, and supported each other's drive to improve. Being part of the team boosted Hannah's self-esteem and gave her structure, an admirable work ethic, an appreciation for fitness, and a close-knit group of friends.

But the sport, which included year-round training (cross-country trained in the summer and fall; track trained in the winter and spring), wasn't without its injuries and strains. Hannah had a number of them, and dealt with intermittent pain after each one.

There was the time she tripped over a tree root the summer before her sophomore year—a summer in which she'd run nearly three hundred miles as part of a team challenge. On that particular day, when she stumbled, she put her leg out in front of her body to keep herself from falling, which caused the top of her thigh bone to jam into her pelvis, injuring her sacrum (the triangular bone at the base of the spine).

The incident triggered intense pain that originated from her sacroiliac (SI) joints—which connect the hip bones to the sacrum— and radiated down her leg. "At first it was really acute and it would hurt when I put any weight on my leg," remembers Hannah. "Then it became a really uncomfortable ache when I would try and run on it." After about two weeks of running while in pain, Hannah realized she had perhaps pushed things too far: "I wouldn't say it was because of my incredible willpower, though. I would say it was just because I was stupid and kept pushing on something that I should have let rest."

That fall, the injury forced Hannah to take a break from cross-country running. A visit to the doctor proved unhelpful, but she got advice from her coach and teammates, and ultimately found relief by resting, biking, icing the area, and seeing a massage therapist who specialized in sports injuries. (Nonsteroidal anti-inflammatory medications like ibuprofen didn't seem to make a big difference in how Hannah felt so she didn't rely on medication.) Her pain lessened after about a month so she returned to the team and went on to have a very successful sophomore season. But her mom, Jill, remembers that "the injury kind of plagued her."

During her junior year, Hannah's SI joint pain came back. "It just started hurting again, so this time I biked until it felt okay to run on," says Hannah, who was sidelined during the beginning of the fall cross-country season for the second year in a row. "I didn't wait until it was completely healed, but this time it went away a lot more quickly because I wasn't trying to run on it."

Throughout high school, in addition to the SI joint pain, Hannah also dealt with twisted ankles, knee strain, tension in her psoas muscle (a muscle that connects the lower back to the thigh via the pelvis), and shin splints, which she would run through—to a point. Over the years, she visited her pediatrician, a podiatrist, an orthotics specialist, an orthopedist, and physical therapists, each of which resulted in little to no relief. Her senior year, Hannah didn't run the spring track season at all. Between the SI joint pain and the shin splints, "running wasn't really satisfying for me right then because it was painful," she says.

Still, Hannah says her injuries have not been a big deal—especially compared to other teammates who have endured breaks and ligament tears, and sports-ending surgeries. After all, Hannah has only had to sit out for portions of seasons, she says, and massage and rest have typically done the trick for her—at least until her pain flares up again.

Ask most young athletes who are serious about their sport and they'll tell you that Hannah's experience is common. For them, training hard is not without sacrifice, and pain is simply a by-product of playing competitively. "I feel like I accept the pain and I work around it," says Hannah. "I cross train, I do other things, and I definitely seek out help for it." Managing acute or chronic pain is just part of the game.

The Surge in Sports Injuries

Participation in youth sports programs is at an all-time high in the United States. Although estimates vary, between thirty million and sixty million children are thought to participate in organized team sports in this country—and competition is fierce. In many cases, parents and kids view excelling in a sport as not merely a way to stay fit and have fun, but also as part of the path to college. The harder kids train and the more forceful they are on the field, the better their chances are of receiving a scholarship or admission into the college of their choice. As a result, young athletes are going full throttle, playing year-round on both school and club teams, participating in travel teams and tournaments, and going to sports camps during off-seasons.

This level of continuous play has led to a sharp increase in injuries. "Kids these days are just playing a lot more than they ever did before, and in some cases more intensely than they ever did before," says Tracy Mehan of the Center for Injury Research and Policy at Nationwide Children's Hospital in Columbus, which has assessed injury rates in youth sports. "All those things will contribute to the increase in injuries."

Nationwide, approximately eight thousand children are treated in emergency rooms *each day* for painful sports-related injuries. Among children under age fourteen, more than 3.5 million receive medical treatment for sports injuries yearly. Among high-school athletes, each year brings two million sports injuries, five hundred thousand doctor visits, and thirty thousand hospitalizations.[1]

Study after study involving youth sports around the country finds soaring rates of injuries such as broken bones, sprains, tears, and lacerations. Concussions—sustained when a blow or jolt to the head causes the brain to jostle within the skull and damages brain cells— have also risen dramatically.

One study published in the journal *Pediatrics* found that among youth soccer players aged seven to seventeen, the decade from 2004 to 2014 saw a 74 percent increase in injuries treated in emergency departments.[2] Another study, by Daniel Green, a pediatric ortho- pedic surgeon at the Hospital for Special Surgery (HSS) in Man- hattan, reveals that in the state of New York in the past twenty years, knee injuries from sports have resulted in a threefold increase in anterior cruciate ligament (ACL) surgeries in children.[3]

Indeed, ACL tears are becoming commonplace around the country among children involved in competitive soccer, lacrosse, basketball, gymnastics, and other sports.[4] Girls are particularly vulnerable to ACL injuries when playing sports, with most research indicating this is due to anatomical, hormonal, and neuromuscular differences, but they are hardly alone.[5] Robert Marx, an orthopedic surgeon at HSS and coauthor of *The ACL Solution: Prevention and Recovery for Sports' Most Devastating Knee Injury,* says that, regardless of gender, "ACL injury is an epidemic; I have performed ACL recon- struction surgery on children as young as seven."

Children's elbows and shoulders are also susceptible to strains and tears, especially when they play sports such as baseball, soft- ball, and tennis, according to the organization STOP Sports Injuries. Case in point: research published in the *American Journal of Sports Medicine* found a dramatic rise in the number of teen baseball pitchers undergoing "Tommy John" surgery, a procedure named after the Major League Baseball pitcher Tommy John which involves replacing a torn or ruptured ligament in the elbow called the ulnar collateral ligament.[6] "Tommy John surgery used to be reserved for college or even high-school-level kids, but now I see the injury in younger and younger kids," says Joshua Dines, an orthopedic surgeon at HSS and associate team physician for the New York Mets, among other professional teams.

"The take-home message is that the actual number of kids who are hurt—that physicians have to take care of—has increased over time, and it's not just because more kids are playing," says Dawn Comstock, a professor of epidemiology at the Colorado School of Public Health who leads the National High School Sports-Related Injury Surveillance Study. Kids are playing more intensely for longer periods of time and for more days out of the year. And the research is showing that their bodies pay the price.

Overzealous and Overused

One of the most significant factors behind the dramatic rise in youth sports injuries is sports specialization. Relative to the past, many more children today concentrate on one sport and play that sport throughout the year. This means they repeat the same movements, using the same muscles and joints, over and over—in, say, five practices a week and ten games a month—with little time off to let the body recuperate. The constant stress on specific areas of the body leads to overuse injuries, such as ligament tears, tendonitis, shin splints (typical among runners like Hannah), and growth plate fractures and breaks. Study after study on patterns in kids' sports-related pain and injuries finds that kids who play a single sport year-round have much higher pain and injury risk than kids who don't play year round. In the case of back pain, it doesn't matter if a young athlete is a football player, gymnast, or wrestler: if they engage in their sport year-round, they nearly double the likelihood they will suffer acute and chronic back pain. In the majority of cases, it's the repetitive movements and overuse of the same areas of the body that lead to painful injuries in children and teens.[7]

"When I grew up, you'd play soccer or football in the fall, you'd play basketball or hockey in the winter, and then you'd play baseball in the spring, maybe into the summer. So just by the nature of the seasons, you'd use different body parts over the year, you'd focus on different things, and you wouldn't be able to play baseball in November and December. Now it's become an all-year sport. And even the Mets know that shouldn't be the case," says Dr. Dines. "Overuse injuries that lead to tendonitis, inflammation, and pain used to get better with rest. But now they're progressing to full tears because kids never get that chance to rest."

Even well-meaning coaches can unknowingly set a child up for an overuse injury. "Many coaches don't realize that a kid is on two or three teams and going to a showcase that weekend," says Daryl Osbahr, managing director and chief of orthopaedic surgery for Rothman Orthopaedic Institute in Florida and a team physician and consultant for numerous professional sports teams. "So, even though each coach may be doing the right thing for that child, the kid might still be making fifty or a hundred more throws than desired because they're doing it in various settings."

There are some team environments, though, that encourage kids to push themselves too far. When Rachel played volleyball in high school, the coach's mantra was "Ball before body!" This meant that players should dive for balls without worrying about bodily harm. The coach surely didn't wish injuries on her players, but if young athletes are consistently taught to sacrifice their body for a save or a point, they are probably more likely to get hurt.

Another factor in the rise in sports injuries is the increasingly aggressive nature of youth sports. Brian Hafter, a girls' youth soccer coach and referee in San Bruno, California, says that the way kids play soccer now is very different from how he and his sister played the game growing up. "There's no question that nowadays the players are much more physical, challenging for the ball," he says, "and, as a result, can put themselves and their opponents in situations that can lead to more serious injuries."

Not surprisingly, youth football has also become more competitive and seen an increase in reported injuries, particularly as concussion awareness has taken center field. In children aged ten to nineteen, there was a 71 percent increase in sports-related concussion between 2010 and 2015, and the peak season for these traumatic brain injuries was fall—when football and rugby are played. Granted, this rise can be partially explained by recent national education efforts to help coaches, parents, and athletes identify the signs of concussion and seek help at emergency departments or urgent care clinics when a concussion is suspected. But experts say that the high incidence of concussion is not merely a product of increased reporting and mandated concussion protocols set forth by sports leagues or states. The high concussion rate is also due in large part to the sheer number of blows that children in contact sports sustain.[8]

"Emergency department data can be an overrepresentation of concussions because parents are so worried about concussions right now that they may take children to the emergency department for a minor concussion when they wouldn't take children to the emergency department for a minor ankle sprain," explains Dr. Comstock, who was one of five experts to speak at the White House in 2014 for the Healthy Kids and Safe Sports Concussion Summit.

"That can skew what we see in data sets and it can sometimes make it look like concussions are a bigger deal than they really are. But make no mistake: concussions are a big deal." (For more on how to handle concussions, see the side bar in this chapter, and the tips in Chapter 7 on headaches.)

The Price of Unacknowledged Pain

Even when young athletes seek help for an injury and visit the emergency department, pain management at the hospital is often suboptimal, which is ironic given that pain is usually what brings them to the doctor. Yet when kids, parents, coaches, and even doctors view the body as something that needs only a mechanical or structural fix, the pain often gets pushed aside and is relegated to being a secondary symptom. And when the pain goes untreated, it tends to linger, which can lead to longer-term suffering.

When young athletes continue playing their sport despite being in pain, they can pay a very high toll. In the early stages of many injuries, full recoveries are possible if children sit out a game or two or take time to rest during off-seasons to give their bodies time to heal. But when a kid doesn't get adequate time to recuperate and rehabilitate, that same injury may be exacerbated, and end up causing a whole season to be missed—or worse, keeping that child from ever returning to play or regaining full physical function.

"When it comes to pain, the first thing I tell parents and kids is that if something hurts they've got to back off, because nothing good comes from playing through the pain," says Dr. Dines. "I tell my professional patients the same thing: this isn't 'no pain, no gain.' Even when parents say their child is only hurting a little and he's still throwing well, that shouldn't be the discussion. Pain is a warning sign for the body that it's being exposed to something that it doesn't want to be exposed to, and playing through it is only risking further injury." (Note that this advice relates to the *acute* pain associated with an injury. In a *chronic* pain condition in which an injury has healed, yet the nervous system has become hypersensitized to pain signals, other guidance applies, as discussed in Chapter 1 and elsewhere.)

Dr. Dines explains that ignoring acute pain can lead either to a larger injury at the site of the discomfort or to dysfunction in a different area as the body tries to compensate and offset the initial pain. "The body is not stupid, so a child may change his delivery a little in throwing or in his serve motion," he says, "and now the body is exposed to another potential injury as it alters its form and puts other ligaments out of alignment."

Things can get even more complicated when injuries require surgery. The younger that kids start with surgery, says Dr. Dines, the lower their chances of long-term success. "If you have your first surgery when you're twelve, and you keep playing, it's almost a foregone conclusion that the injury and surgery is going to happen again when you're seventeen or eighteen, and then again at age twenty-five—and you've just shifted the timeline back, which is a bigger problem," he explains. "The reason for this is that, anytime you start operating on the same body part multiple times, the results typically aren't as good and I'm not very optimistic that you're going to keep doing well."[9]

Life-Long Consequences

Hannah's mother, Jill, knows firsthand how a sports injury can alter the course of a life, because it happened to her when she was a young track athlete. "In middle school, I was running over the finish line during a track meet—running as fast as I ever ran before or since—and I ripped all the tendons in my ankle. And, I'll admit it, I continued to play sports. I didn't continue track, but I played soccer throughout junior year," says Jill. "The trainer would tape my ankle for the game, and afterward, when the tape was cut off, I'd frequently sprain my ankle stepping off a curb or out of a car. Many severe sprains caused me to spend an inordinate amount of my teen years on crutches. It also caused me to develop a lot of physical fear."

Jill had ankle reconstructive surgery between her junior and senior year, and decided then that it was best to leave athletics behind in favor of theater and student government. "That one surgery changed my whole life," she says.

But Jill's physical issues didn't end there. In her mid-forties, she developed chronic hip pain that led her to walk with a cane and, when the aching was too severe for her to sleep, to take Celebrex (a prescription nonsteroidal anti-inflammatory drug). She was diagnosed with hip dysplasia and underwent hip replacement surgery at age fifty-one. "I think I was compensating for my ankle and walking strangely, which may have altered my gait and caused my right hip to deteriorate faster," says Jill. "But I have my life back from this surgery." Still, it was a long and painful journey that had started nearly forty years earlier, with a middle-school sports injury.

Anna sees many adolescent patients starting down this same road. For a number of them, what started out as a minor athletic injury has developed into a problem that, if it is not addressed effectively, threatens to be life-long. Like Jill and her daughter, these patients expected that the pain from their sports injuries would be short-lived. But more often than people realize, the pain from these sorts of injuries persists, and sometimes spreads. The children who come to see Anna and other members of the pediatric pain management team where she works have already seen their pediatricians, and typically, beyond that, they've worked with orthopedists, rheumatologists, physical therapists, massage therapists, and other specialists. They have missed weeks of school and had to step away from sports they love. Between this and the irritability that so often comes with experiencing persistent pain, their mood has also taken a nosedive.

Why Sports Injuries Become Chronic Pain Problems

One of Anna's colleagues, Amy L. Holley, a psychologist and associate professor at Oregon Health and Science University, is trying to solve the mystery of why the pain from acute musculoskeletal injuries (like sprains and broken bones) sometimes fails to resolve. Dr. Holley's studies are among the first to evaluate children with acute musculoskeletal injuries and follow them over time. One paper (which Anna coauthored) reports on the experience of children with broken bones, sprains, and other injuries to muscles or ligaments (many from sports injuries) in the four months after their initial visits to emergency departments and outpatient clinics. The goal of the research was to identify physiological, psychological, and behavioral factors that might predict which kids would recover and bounce back from their injuries and which kids would develop chronic pain.

The first findings were that about 35 percent of children who came in with acute musculoskeletal pain continued to experience pain four months after their initial doctor's visit, and notably, these children were much more likely to be girls. In fact, of the kids with persistent pain, more than 87 percent were girls, and less than 13 percent were boys.

Another striking discovery: kids were just as likely to have pain four months later whether they had a relatively minor injury or a major broken bone.

So, what factors predicted whose pain endured? Dr. Holley's research team found clues by looking at each child's conditioned pain modulation (CPM), which is a person's inherent ability to dampen or inhibit pain in response to particular stimuli (and is part of the descending pain pathway in the nervous system, as explained in Chapter 1). It is possible to measure CPM in the lab by exposing a person to certain conditions and evaluating how their body responds. In this study, each child participated in such an exercise soon after their first visit to the doctor, and researchers used heat and cold stimuli to assess how the child's pain modulation system was working. What they found four months after injury was that children whose pain modulation systems had been working efficiently at the outset were more likely to have recovered and be pain-free. Meanwhile, children who had higher depressive symptoms around the time of their injury were more likely to be disabled by their pain four months later. These results support the idea that nervous system functioning and mood are important influences in pain responses—perhaps even as important as the severity of the injury itself. We still don't know whether it's possible to change or improve a person's conditioned pain modulation system—or whether improving it would improve overall pain outcomes—but these are questions that researchers hope to explore in the future.[10]

The Upside to Sports Participation

Now for the good news about sports and pain: While sports participation comes with inherent risks for injury, research also suggests that playing sports responsibly and being generally active may lower children's risk for developing chronic pain problems. For instance, in some studies, teens who participate in organized sports, such as swimming and soccer, have a decreased risk of developing lower back pain, and kids who spend more time sitting have an increased risk.[11] One large study done in Norway revealed that teenagers who exercised rigorously several days a week had lower risk for chronic pain problems than teens who exercised fewer days per week.[12]

Why would *more* activity lead to *less* pain? Studies in the general population have long shown that moderate physical activity boosts health and well-being. Meanwhile, researchers focusing on elite athletes have been looking into how intense physical activity affects perception of pain. Lab experiments have found that, when athletes are exposed to painful stimuli like heat, pressure, and cold, their tolerance for the sensations is higher than that of non-athletes. And this higher threshold for pain may be due to psychological factors, according to a study of ultra-marathon runners. In this research (which included a lab-based test and a questionnaire), the runners exhibited less pain-related anxiety and less pain avoidance than the non-runners. It's as if the experience of running very long distances had taught them to focus less on pain as an alarm or as a true threat to their bodies.[13]

Other studies have assessed trained athletes through neuroimaging and found that regular physical activity can change how our brains process painful stimuli and affect how we perceive that pain. Findings like this suggest a role for exercise in both prevention and treatment of chronic pain.[14]

Setting a Steady Pace

It was a hot and humid September day in Massachusetts when Hannah and hundreds of other cross-country runners from high schools around New England gathered to compete in a 5K race. Jill and her husband, Matt, were standing near the finish line waiting for Hannah to emerge from the wooded trail. But first, they watched the varsity boys come through—a pack of bodies speeding over the finish line.

"The boys were running so fast that they were running into each other," Jill recalls. "They had really strong volunteers, parents, and coaches standing there at the finish line to grab the kids when they came through to slow them down and hold them up—because a lot of them would fall down after they'd exerted every ounce of their energy."

Hannah usually didn't show signs of distress, but on this day, with temperatures in the nineties, she reached a breaking point. "When Hannah came over the line, she had really pushed it, and she blacked out and fainted," says Jill. "My friend was working the finish line and she literally caught Hannah mid-fall and brought her over to the medical tent."

Hannah quickly regained consciousness in the tent but her parents were alarmed by what they saw happening around them. "There were girls throwing up and crying, and others were sitting there with ice packs and wet towels on their heads," remembers Jill. "My husband and I were watching this, and he looked at me and said, 'I don't want her to run anymore. That's it. I think we should forbid it.' So many of these girls were running through injuries and, as a parent, my husband and I often felt like it wasn't worth it, and we were concerned about Hannah's long-term health." Yet, as they learned, striking a balance between healthy competition and overexertion can be highly problematic for parents and young athletes.

Many families grapple with figuring out appropriate limits for their children's sports participation. In Hannah's case, her parents did not end up forbidding her to run. Hannah continued running throughout high school—and went on to compete on her college's Division III cross-country and track teams, and was co-captain of its cross country team her senior year. She wouldn't have done it any differently. "I loved running in high school. I never found it to be an unhealthy thing for me. It gave me a lot of self-confidence," she says. Although her SI joint pain kicks into high gear every now and then, for Hannah, the rewards of her sport far outweighed the pain.

"Parenting is a long, slow process of letting your kids go and letting them make their own independent choices," explains Jill. "So my thought process was to continue to communicate with Hannah about how the most important thing is not to win; the most important things are to be healthy and strong and feel great about yourself." She hopes Hannah will heed that message and feel empowered by running for a lifetime; and if her pain flares, she'll listen to her body and adapt as needed.

Injury Prevention and Treatment

Fortunately, with appropriate training techniques, adequate time off, and the guidance of knowledgeable adults, young athletes can up their chances of preventing sports injuries from happening in the first place. And when injuries do happen, there are steps kids can take to minimize long-term problems.

To keep a young athlete strong, happy, and healthy (both mentally and physically), talk with potential coaches about their approach and keep in mind these recommendations from experts, including the American Academy of Pediatrics:

- Help your child adopt a healthy mindset. In many sports, children are mentally conditioned to brush off pain and discomfort to their detriment. "There is the idea that you must sacrifice your body and your brain for the overall greater good of the team," says Dawson Dicks, a football coach in the Boston area who has worked with high school and college teams. He acknowledges that this mentality can be taken too far. Whether your child's sport is football, track, soccer, or volleyball, your basic advice should be the same: "listen to your body. Take time to recover when you're hurt." The longer a child plays injured, the more likely it is that chronic problems will develop.

· Make prevention a priority. Fewer injuries mean fewer opportunities for nervous system function to go haywire. But keep in mind that prevention doesn't just mean physical stretching and strength training. It also means helping children reduce stress and get enough sleep. We know that both mental well-being and adequate rest have the potential to protect children from developing persistent pain—and that many of the kids and parents driven to excessive athletic participation also feel enormous pressure to excel at academics and in other areas. When this competitive environment costs kids sleep, it puts both their physical and mental health at risk.

· Delay sports specialization until at least age fifteen (better yet, sixteen) to minimize stress on your child's growing body and decrease the likelihood of overuse injuries. Encouraging a kid to play a variety of sports throughout the year helps to strengthen different muscles and reduces the chances of burning out on just one activity.

- Make sure young athletes take two days off from their sport every week throughout the season to lower the likelihood of overuse injuries. This doesn't mean kids must be inactive on their days off. They can, for instance, go swimming on their days away from the softball field.
- Encourage kids to take time away from their main sport for at least three months during the year, in installments of one month. During that time, kids should try other physical activities, or stay active by playing outside and having fun with friends.
- Closely supervise a young athlete who does specialize in a single sport. Ideally, team up with your child's pediatrician and a coach or knowledgeable athletic trainer to provide appropriate guidance.
- Teach children to seek help when they are in pain. Pain is the body's best way of alerting them that they should stop what they are doing and reassess.
- Maintain sight of long-term goals. If the hope is that a person will be physically active for the rest of his life, pushing the body to its limit during every youthful game may backfire. "We want to encourage all young athletes to give maximum effort and be competitive," says Dr. Osbahr, "but we also always need to encourage them to achieve their ultimate goals with the ideals of health and safety in mind."
- Seek out teams that have athletic trainers. Not to be confused with coaches, athletic trainers are healthcare professionals who work under the direction of doctors and can provide athletes with proper conditioning, injury

prevention, and rehabilitation. Having licensed athletic trainers on the field can also be vital in emergency situations.

· Urge athletes to respect the rules of the game to lower the chances of dangerous plays. "One of the things parents can do to keep their kids safe is make sure that your kid's coach is insisting upon fair play and good sportsmanship, and make sure that whatever league your child is playing in has qualified refs who enforce the rules," says Dr. Comstock. "If the vast majority of athlete-to-athlete contact were restricted according to the rules of the game, we'd have less concussion as well as fewer other injuries," she says.

· Ask coaches what they do to prevent injury and keep young athletes safe. For instance, if a football coach is teaching blocking, find out about his training and technique. "If you don't have the expertise to teach young kids how to go about doing something as serious as tackling, you could get a whole lot of kids hurt," says Dicks. If you have concerns about the coaches or adults in charge, speak up.

· Find out about conditioning programs. For example, to reduce the risk of ACL injuries, Dr. Marx recommends injury-prevention programs that target core and hip strength, body position, balance, and movement patterns. Ask the athletic trainer, coach, or pediatrician about safe strategies.

· Check in with your child regularly. Playing sports can be a boon for a child's mental well-being. It can foster discipline, improved self-esteem, goal-setting abilities, and leadership skills. It can also teach kids about the importance and the joy of working with a team. But pressure to excel or win, if it becomes too intense, can chip away at the psychological benefits of sports participation. That's why parents and coaches would be wise to ask children periodically if they're still feeling motivated and enjoying their sport. Just as there is a need to have a healthy balance between physical training and periods of rest, it's important for kids to have a healthy balance between sports competition and playing for fun.

What to do when an injury happens:

- If an injury does develop, seek medical care, and make sure your child takes the time off that's needed to truly recover. Often this will include physical therapy. "I always emphasize the value of rest," says Barbara Bergin, an orthopedic surgeon in Austin and cofounder of Texas Orthopedics, Sports, and Rehabilitation Associates. "Nobody wants to rest. They want to take pain-relieving medications and be able to go to school or work. But I suggest that, if you need a pain pill, then you should stay home and rest. With children, I focus on lots of ice, elevation, and TLC."

- If surgery is required, help your child be realistic about the amount of time it means out of the game and find other ways to stay busy. Dr. Bergin, whose own son was sidelined from football due to serious injuries, advises other young athletes to "do something else that gets your focus off of the sadness of your injury—whether that's a hobby, volunteering, or anything else you enjoy." And, she adds, "if you're planning to return to the sport, try to stay involved while you're recovering by attending practices and games so that you don't lose contact with your teammates and friends."

· If surgery is involved, ask your child's physician about what to expect in terms of recovery. The goal is to use the injured part of the body as much as is feasible and to gradually strengthen it under the supervision of medical professionals. So be prepared with concrete questions: When can my child put weight on the injured area? When should my child expect to resume everyday activities? When will my child be given clearance to exercise and start physical therapy?

· If your child's physician prescribes pain medication, be clear on how many days it needs to be taken, and whether over-the-counter (OTC) pain medications can be used simultaneously. In some cases, children can start off with a lower dose of prescription pain medication if they combine it with an OTC pain reliever approved by the doctor. Prescription pain medications are often prescribed with no instructions about when or how to stop using them. If one is likely to be needed for more than a few days, ask your child's physician how to taper the dose or frequency.

· If your child's mood is erratic, take note. Some irritability and moodiness is a normal part of teenage life, but if you have any concern about your child's state of mind, don't be afraid to talk about it: seek input from your pediatrician, a behavioral health provider (many pediatrician's offices now have these professionals on staff), or a school counselor. A positive mood can help with injury recovery.

· If recovery seems to be taking a long time, ask the doctor about reasonable expectations. Recovery does take time, so it's important to be aware that physical capabilities won't return overnight, and that it may take considerable effort to get back into pre-injury shape. Be as positive as possible about the hard work your child is doing. Celebrate your child's progress toward a healthy recovery just as you would celebrate scoring a goal or winning a game. Cheer on your young athlete every step of the way.

Heads Up: When in Doubt, Sit Them Out

Despite today's enhanced focus on concussions in young athletes and in professional athletes—especially those in the National Football League and National Hockey League—adolescent players still often ignore the nausea, dizziness, headaches, and sensitivity to light that are well-known symptoms of a head injury.

"Kids are often reluctant to acknowledge a concussion because they may want a scholarship for college, or their dad or coach wants them to play, or they want to get back on the field and do their part—so they may be a little dishonest about what they're truly feeling," says football coach Dicks. But acknowledging and treating pain and injury in the moment is crucial—particularly when there is a suspected concussion.

Research published in the journal *Pediatrics* shows that kids who suffer a concussion and continue to play sports in the minutes afterward take nearly twice as long to recover as the children who leave the game immediately after a head trauma. In the study, conducted through the Sports Medicine Concussion Program at the University of Pittsburgh Medical Center, thirty-five teenage athletes (who came from football, soccer, ice hockey, volleyball, field hockey, basketball, wrestling, and rugby) were taken out of the game right after getting a concussion, as is protocol for concussion treatment. Their experience was compared to a separate group of thirty-four athletes who had sustained concussions but remained on the field and continued playing. The researchers found that the players who stayed in the game after head trauma took an average of forty-four days to recover, while the athletes who left the game immediately required only an average of twenty-two days.[15]

The implication is that a period of rest of twenty-four to forty-eight hours after a concussion—followed by a gradual return to normal activities under the supervision of a doctor—allows brain cells to heal faster. "When the brain is concussed, that network of neurons within the brain are not communicating well with each other. Further physical activity or further cognitive exertion further stresses the system," says Tad Seifert, a neurologist and director of the Sports Concussion Program for Norton Healthcare, in Louisville, Kentucky.

Additionally, as compared to adults, adolescents are more vulnerable to the physiological effects of concussion because their brains are still developing, explains R. J. Elbin, who led the *Pediatrics* study while at the University of Pittsburgh. Elbin, now director of the Office for Sport Concussion Research at the University of Arkansas, points to advice by the US Centers for Disease Control and Prevention—"When in doubt, sit them out" and "It's better to miss one game than the rest of the season"—and he adds that "our data supports that." The lesson: players, coaches, trainers, and parents need to be aware of the signs of concussion and immediately test athletes for a suspected head injury following a blow.

Taking a break after a concussion is essential, but it's also true that resting for too long can be problematic. In one study, researchers at the Medical College of Wisconsin randomly assigned children who were diagnosed with mild concussions to two different treatment groups. In one group, families were told by the doctor that the child needed to rest for one to two days before gradually returning to normal activities; in the other group, the doctor ordered strict rest (no physical activity, school, or work) for five days. In check-ins ten days after the injury, the kids who were told to rest for five days reported *higher* levels of post-concussive symptoms (like headaches and dizziness) than the kids who were prescribed the shorter rest period. This simple difference in what a physician prescribed impacted how the children recovered over time.[16]

What else can be done to improve outcomes? Studies show that when children and parents have accurate information about concussion recovery and are given appropriate advice on how to gradually return to normal activities, kids recover from headaches and other concussion symptoms more quickly.[17] Research also reveals that kids recover faster when they receive collaborative care that includes psychological and behavioral interventions (such as cognitive behavioral therapy) alongside treatment from sports medicine providers, rehabilitation specialists, and neurologists.[18] Still, while the average recovery time from sports-related concussion in ten- to seventeen-year-olds is seventeen days, about one quarter of these kids still struggle with symptoms more than a month after their injury.[19] Much remains to be discovered about concussion treatment. (For more specific guidance on concussions, see Chapter 5 on headaches.)

Chapter 9

Pain as a Disease State

*When the nervous system goes awry—
and how to correct course*

For decades, we assumed that if someone was in persistent pain, it must be the result of an underlying anatomical condition. Doctors and patients alike believed that pain in the muscles or bones (known as musculoskeletal pain) had to be caused by physical trauma (like a strained muscle), infection (like an earache), or ongoing chronic disease (like cancer). What was needed for the pain to go away, they thought, was to treat the underlying condition. In recent years, however, researchers have discovered that this assumption doesn't always hold true. There are some diseases of which pain is both the primary symptom and the underlying condition. In these cases, even if the pain was triggered by an injury or illness, the pain doesn't dissipate when the initial condition is treated. Instead, the nervous system becomes hypersensitized, causing the pain to linger and intensify—often with no physical clues of its origin—saddling families with a maddening mystery. But pain researchers and clinicians have become wise to this phenomenon and have begun to classify this type of chronic pain as a disease state in and of itself.

Remember Taylor, from this book's introduction? At almost nine years old, she developed one such condition, called complex regional pain syndrome (CRPS)—also known as reflex sympathetic dystrophy—after a classmate rolled over her foot while they were roller-skating. The accident didn't cause a sprain, break, or other obvious injury, yet Taylor endured more than a year and a half of debilitating pain because her nervous system went into overdrive. And while physicians struggled to identify a clear cause for her pain, that didn't make it any less real. Fortunately, Taylor received intensive treatment for CRPS which lessened her pain significantly. Now in high school, she does continue to have pain flares but has learned how to manage her symptoms.

In this chapter, we'll focus on CRPS and also on juvenile-onset fibromyalgia, which is characterized by widespread pain, fatigue, and sleep disturbances. Both are pain-driven conditions involving a hypersensitive nervous system and, because they are frequently misunderstood, both often go undiagnosed and untreated for months or years. But scientists have done substantial recent work to decipher these conditions. They've delved into the neurobiology of these diseases, and discovered that they are caused by changes in peripheral nerve function (affecting nerves in the feet and hands and other extremities), and in how the central nervous system handles pain signals (a process that takes place in the spinal cord and brain). This improved understanding of what may be causing the pain is enabling practitioners to better treat it.

Complex Regional Pain Syndrome: Tyler's Story

Imagine for a moment that someone is stroking your arm with a feather but, instead of feeling a light tickle, you feel as if you are being burned by a hot torch. A gust of wind feels like a knife cutting your skin. The touch of your cotton T-shirt or bedsheet feels like a million needles piercing your body. In short, you feel excruciating pain even though there is no harmful, external trigger. These examples, says Elliot Krane, chief of pain management at the Packard Children's Hospital and professor of anesthesiology at Stanford University Medical Center, give you an inkling of what it feels like to have CRPS.

The condition, affecting about two hundred thousand people in the United States in any given year, typically begins with a relatively minor injury, such as a sprained ankle or a broken wrist, which triggers pain. Under normal circumstances, after a physical trauma like that, treatments that may include rest, ice, anti-inflammatory medication, a short period of immobilization (a cast or a splint), and perhaps physical therapy, the injury heals and the nervous system calms down. But for 7 to 10 percent of people, after the injury resolves, the nervous system doesn't recalibrate and it does not return to its previous "normal" set point.[1] Instead, the nerves stay switched on and go into overdrive, sending constant pain signals to the brain even though there may be no physical trace of the original injury.

That's what happened to Tyler, of Queens, New York, when he was twelve years old. In April of 2015, after a mishap on a stationary bike, Tyler broke his ankle and a bone in his foot. He was given an orthopedic boot to immobilize the area, and although his bones healed, he began to develop a limp. Later that year, in September, he fell while zip-lining, and broke his ankle and foot in the same places. Again, Tyler wore a boot on his foot, but this time, his bones didn't heal easily, so the orthopedist gave him a cast. Eventually, his bones healed. But when his cast was removed, his foot looked discolored and he felt even more pain.

"He was crying in pain at night and he couldn't walk on his foot during the day," says his mother, Denise. But because an MRI showed only inflammation around the foot and ankle, the orthopedist concluded that there was nothing wrong and that Tyler must be faking his complaints to get out of school. "This was a studious boy, a straight-A student who loved school, and I knew that wasn't the case," Denise says.

In their search for treatment, in November 2015, Denise took Tyler to a physical therapist. By then, Tyler's foot had become purple, swollen, and cold (all classic signs of CRPS)—and he couldn't bear for it to be touched. The physical therapist was the first practitioner to recognize the symptoms of CRPS that Tyler was experiencing and suggest that he might have the condition.

"This kid was in constant pain, twenty-four/seven. He could barely sleep at times. I'd hear him banging on the wall at night because of the pain; and to hear the moans, it was very, very difficult," says Denise. Even simple tasks became nearly insurmountable. For instance, Tyler couldn't handle the sensation of water on his foot, so showering became an ordeal. "It was heartbreaking what he went through."

Denise also remembers how hard it was for other people to understand what was happening. After all, pain is not a shared experience, and only the person feeling the pain can truly know its impact. Even Tyler's dad had to see it to believe it. As a way of verifying that the pain was real, Denise says that Tyler's dad "would wait until Tyler was sleeping to touch his foot lightly and then he would see that, even in his sleep, Tyler winced from the pain."

In December 2015, a pediatric orthopedist confirmed that Tyler had CRPS. But as with many people who face chronic pain syndromes, it took nearly a year for the family to find a pediatric pain specialist who had expertise in this area and had availability to see them. At its worst, by January 2016, the discoloration had extended up Tyler's leg, his leg muscles had become dystonic (tending to contract involuntarily), he was using a walker to get around, and he needed to be home-schooled. He'd tried the medications gabapentin (a generic drug often prescribed to treat seizures and nerve pain) and Lyrica (a brand-name drug also used to treat seizures and nerve pain)—both medications that can be effective for some people. For Tyler, however, they only made things worse. "The medications made him violent. There were times he would be screaming bloody murder and I would have to try to hold him down to help him relax," says Denise.

At one point, in a frantic attempt to get her son some relief, Denise took Tyler to the emergency department. He was admitted for three days and given the medications tramadol, morphine, and oxycodone (all opioids), but nothing took away the pain.

Finally, the family got an appointment with a pediatric anesthesiologist who understood CRPS and knew how to help. "Everything changed when we found her," says Denise. The doctor helped wean Tyler off the medication he was taking and instead recommended a two-pronged approach: a physical therapist who specialized in CRPS and a psychologist who focused on treating pain with cognitive behavioral therapy. It was a long road and required an enormous amount of work and perseverance, but slowly, Tyler's condition began to improve. A turning point came in July 2016, when the family attended a week-long family camp for children with CRPS run by the US Pain Foundation. "It was very powerful to interact with other children and parents dealing with the same thing. We thought we were the only ones," says Denise. "Camp changed his whole way of life. My nonathlete has run three Spartan races in the last three years, and he's been pain-free since November 2016." Tyler, now a junior in high school, has kept his grade point average up, and has set his sights on becoming an orthopedic surgeon. "I'm so grateful for where we are now. It did not come easy—we had to push and fight for it—but we got here," says Denise. "Now, Tyler's doctors have their new patients' parents call me to help them through and give them hope."

Making Sense of a Mysterious Disease

"How can the nervous system get it so wrong?" asks Dr. Krane in a widely viewed TED talk that Anna often recommends to her patients. "How can the nervous system misinterpret an innocent sensation like the touch of a feather, and turn it into the touch of a flame?"[2] As discussed in Chapter 1, our nerve endings respond to sensations by sending chemical messages (via neurotransmitters) up through the spinal cord to the brain, where the messages are interpreted. Once the sensation is decoded, the brain sends messages back down the spinal cord, which may increase or decrease pain levels. But in the case of CRPS, the central nervous system gets hypersensitized and continues sending signals up and down the pain pathway even after the initial injury has healed.

Researchers are still figuring out the multifaceted reasons why the central nervous system becomes sensitized, but one important contributing factor that's been identified in recent years is the role of glial cells within the central nervous system. Scientists have found that the neurotransmitters traveling up and down the pain pathway can activate glial cells, which release chemicals that cause nerve inflammation. And this neuroinflammatory response is part of what tricks the nervous system into misconstruing the stroke of a feather as the burn of fire.[3]

Risk Factors for CRPS

Why does CRPS develop in some people and not in others? Why does one child break her arm and recover in a matter of weeks while another child's injury turns into chronic, debilitating pain? Scientists have identified several factors that seem to make kids more prone to CRPS. "The origins of these chronic pain problems are quite complex and can be biological, genetic, infectious, epigenetic, and there can be a zillion different things that go into the mix to create the central sensitization," says Neil Schechter, director of the Chronic Pain Clinic at Boston Children's Hospital and associate professor of anesthesiology at Harvard Medical School.[4]

There are, though, some clear-cut risk factors for CRPS. For example, age and gender seem to be major players in this condition. The majority of children who develop CRPS do so between the ages of nine and fifteen (the average age of onset is twelve years old), and about 85 percent of the kids diagnosed with CRPS are girls.[5] This has led researchers to believe that hormonal changes associated with puberty may lead adolescent girls to be particularly vulnerable to the condition.

CRPS also seems to be influenced by psychological stressors. Evidence shows that CRPS is more likely to occur when a kid is dealing with a psychiatric condition such as anxiety or depression. A child with CRPS is also more likely to have experienced a stressful event at home (a divorce in the household, for example, or a parent's job change) in the months prior to the onset of their condition.[6] Tyler's mom, Denise, firmly believes that her own medical issues (which landed her in the hospital twice shortly before Tyler developed CRPS) caused a great deal of trauma in their family and contributed to Tyler's condition.

How an injury is treated can also play a role in the development of CRPS—and unlike age, gender, or genetics, this is a factor we have some control over. For instance, research shows that excessive immobilization after an injury can contribute to CRPS.[7] Experiments have even shown that placing a cast on a non-injured arm can cause neurobiological changes that resemble CRPS. In one experiment, a group of adults had casts placed on non-injured forearms for four weeks while a control group of adults did not. When the casts were removed, and for some days later, these adults showed more sensitivity to temperature, pressure on the skin, and normal arm movements—and they even showed discoloration and hair growth changes, all of which are seen in CRPS.[8] Another experiment involving people who volunteered to have their non-injured arm cast for six weeks showed similar results, indicating that treating fractures and sprains with lengthy immobilization may not be the best approach.[9]

Granted, for most people, after a cast is removed from their arm, they spend a few days recalibrating to the renewed stimulation in the environment, and within a week, their nerves return to their pre-injury set point. But for a minority of people, a prolonged lack of nerve stimulation spurs the nervous system to amplify its receptors, causing even mild sensations to register at higher levels. This can signal the beginning of CRPS, particularly if the nervous system is already dealing with other stressors.

Treating CRPS: Retraining the Nervous System, Unlearning Fear

We've learned, then, that the nervous system can overreact to its environment dramatically. On the plus side, though, this illustrates that the nervous system has tremendous plasticity—and we can use this to our advantage. If we slowly expose the nerves to increasing amounts of stimuli, the nervous system can reacclimate and recalibrate. We can retrain our nervous system to get used to sensations if we give it a chance.

In fact, we do this all the time, both in the short term and in the long term. For instance, each time you step into a cold swimming pool, it feels slightly unbearable. But after spending a few minutes in the water, your nervous system usually adapts and you no longer experience the water as too cold. That's a short-term adaptation. On the opposite end of the temperature spectrum, when you first learn how to cook and begin handling warm pots and pans, they feel too hot to touch, which is your nervous system warning you that the stimuli may be dangerous. But after years of mini-exposures to piping hot containers, your nervous system gets used to the sensation, so it no longer sounds a code red alert when you pick up a warm serving platter without oven mitts. "In that scenario, the nervous system has turned down the amplifier," says Dr. Krane. It's essentially signaling, "Okay, I'm telling you this hurts, but if you're not going to listen to me, I'm going to stop telling you." In an experienced chef, the nervous system has recalibrated and changed its "normal" setting to include "hot dishes."

This gradual exposure and eventual acclimation to stimuli is how physical therapists treat CRPS. And it works. "What we do with physical therapy is to give patients a new normal—and it's torture at first, but ultimately we retrain the nerves to respond normally to the activities and sensory experiences that are part of everyday life," says Dr. Krane. The key is to teach children that the chronic pain they feel isn't a protective signal that should stop them from moving. With this type of chronic pain, the nervous system is overreacting and sending unreliable messages about a perceived danger that is not actually a threat. So physical therapists work with kids to do simple tasks—like put weight on their foot for five seconds three times a day—even though they will hurt at first.

"We tell patients that chronic pain hurts but it doesn't harm you," says Dr. Schechter at Boston Children's Hospital. Once kids know that their chronic pain is not an edict to stop moving entirely, they usually have an easier time returning to some of their daily tasks, and moving through the pain despite the extreme discomfort.

Still, overcoming the fear of chronic pain, even if you know an action won't physically harm you, is no small feat. Pain is a very effective teacher; and kids living with the agony of CRPS quickly learn to avoid any movement or situation that might provoke pain's wrath. For many children with CRPS, the mere thought of using their affected limb or of someone at school inadvertently brushing against it is terrifying. That's where psychological tools can help. Cognitive behavioral therapy can help children calm their minds, settle their physiologic state (for instance, by lowering heart rate), and dispel anxiety related to their pain. Using its relaxation and distraction techniques, whether in a physical therapy session or while performing daily tasks, kids can learn to focus less on the pain signals that are generated by their movements and focus more on positive thoughts and images. For example, turning exercises into engaging games or doing them while watching funny videos can distract kids from the immediate pain and fear they may feel while they get their limbs moving. Ideally, a child's treatment plan should not be limited to physical therapy but should also incorporate this kind of cognitive behavioral therapy—and, for that matter, other multidisciplinary strategies such as biofeedback, hypnosis, aromatherapy, and massage. (These approaches are covered in more detail in Chapter 10.)

Remarkably, neuroimaging shows that the connections within children's brains can actually change as a result of these treatments. Research led by Laura Simons, an associate professor of anesthesiology and pediatric pain medicine at Stanford University, has focused on the amygdala, an area of the brain involved in processing fear, anxiety, and memory. She's found that in a young CRPS patient who completes a multidisciplinary rehabilitation program, the amygdala adjusts how it communicates with other parts of the brain. In one study, she compared a group of children with CRPS to a group of children without the condition. "Before treatment started, there was more of the heightened connectivity, or cross-talk, with the amygdala and other areas of the brain in children with CRPS compared to their healthy peers," she says. "What was really exciting is that at the end of treatment—which involved psychology, physical therapy, and occupational therapy—we saw that hyper-connectivity began to dampen down in our patients, and those changes were associated with decreases in pain-related fear." In a matter of weeks, the children's brains responded to the treatment.[10]

Returning to "Normal"

One of the most critical—and low-tech—ways to retrain the nervous system is to resume normal life. But this doesn't mean that kids should power through excruciating pain and jump back to full speed. Returning to normal should be a gradual process. It could mean having your child get out of bed each day to get dressed and sit at the kitchen table for an hour to do a little reading or schoolwork. After a week or two of that level of activity, you might add in a brief daily trip to school, even if it's just to check in with a counselor or homeroom teacher for fifteen minutes. Coupled with a multidisciplinary treatment plan, this slow and steady approach can help kids get back to full functioning.

While timelines for recovery from CRPS vary from person to person, a child in an intensive CRPS program could expect to start seeing real results within a month or so. "Your pain might not disappear, but your function will be improved. Then, over the course of a period of time, your pain should gradually dissipate, and take up less and less space in your life," says Dr. Schechter. "We're extremely optimistic with chronic pain in kids because their nervous systems are very malleable." While some children may have flares or recurrences of CRPS in the months after treatment, about 80 to 90 percent of kids fully recover.[11]

Can Medication Help Treat CRPS?

A large number of the medications that doctors prescribe to children battling chronic pain have not been approved by the Food and Drug Administration for that particular condition or age group. This is called off-label drug prescribing, and it's a common occurrence in medicine. In the field of pediatric pain specifically, it tends to happen for two reasons: few pharmaceutical studies include children, so when seeking options, doctors often turn to medications that have been tested only in adults; and in practice, physicians have often seen a medication prove effective for a condition other than the one it was developed to treat.

For kids with CRPS, in their quest for relief, they are typically prescribed a succession of pain-relieving medications like non-steroidal anti-inflammatory drugs, anti-seizure medications, and opioids. But as in Tyler's experience, those medications are often not very effective in treating this type of pain. While anti-seizure medications such as gabapentin can lessen pain in some children, and antidepressants may also alleviate certain pain conditions, there is little data available on the safety or effectiveness of these medications for treating pain in children. The drugs can also have mood-altering side effects, as they did for Tyler. It has also been widely established that opioids are not the long-term answer for this type of pain. While they may make a teenager with chronic pain less anxious, they're not necessarily going to alleviate the pain. "It takes far too much opioid to make somebody comfortable," explains Dr. Krane, "and you wind up with more mood variability." Of course, opioids are also highly addictive. For all of these reasons, if you're considering pain medication for your child, it's crucial to work closely with a pediatric pain physician to come up with an individualized approach to treatment.

CRPS and Hope for the Future

The more we learn about CRPS in children, the more we may be able to prevent it from becoming severe—or from happening in the first place. We know, for instance, that if a child's pain persists even after a relatively minor injury appears to have healed, it's critical to take that pain seriously. The sooner parents and clinicians address that persistent pain, the easier it is to keep it from snowballing into something bigger. We also know that minimizing time in a cast or a boot, helping adolescents cope with stress, and encouraging children to stay engaged in school and hobbies following an injury are all ways to lessen pain and reduce the fear of pain. The more that parents and clinicians become aware of and act on these strategies, the greater the odds that an isolated injury will be just that—an isolated injury—rather than a trigger for the development of a chronic pain condition.

Juvenile-Onset Fibromyalgia: Sharon's Story

When Sharon Waldrop thinks back on her early years growing up in a suburb of Detroit, she suspects that the symptoms of fibromyalgia began when she was in elementary school, even though doctors didn't label it as such at the time. "I remember intermittently getting a lot of severe pains in my knees, chest, and back, and I was fatigued," says Sharon, who is now in her late forties. "It wasn't the average bump-on-the-knee type of pain, and it scared me. But the pediatrician always told us it was growing pains."

Sharon says that the pain would come and go, and therefore didn't overshadow her childhood, but when it did flare up, she would simultaneously feel sharp pangs and deep aching across her muscles that would last for hours. "I remember it developed out of nowhere—there was no injury—and it became more of a problem at night," she says. "I don't know if I had more willpower during the day or if by nighttime I was worn down and didn't have the ability to deal with it then, but I remember my mom comforting me at bedtime." To try to ease Sharon's pain, her mom would rub Sharon's back, place hot compresses on her body, and give her the occasional Tylenol, but those were the only tactics they had—and they weren't very effective.

Sharon and her mother trusted what the pediatrician told them: these were just "growing pains" and she would have to ride them out. So that's what Sharon tried to do when the pain presented itself. She held it together during the day as much as she could—she didn't miss school—but at nighttime, the pain overtook her body.

By age fifteen, Sharon began having extremely painful menstrual periods. "I felt like I had a ball inside of me that was radiating pain, but the doctors didn't suspect anything was wrong throughout most of my teenage years," she says. "They told me that all women have tough periods and I should just toughen up." But by the time Sharon was off to college at Wayne State University, and she found herself bedridden several days of the week, she knew something was not right. "It was a somewhat traumatic time in college, going it on my own, trying to find a doctor who could help, and going to appointments where they would examine my private parts—I'd feel so vulnerable," remembers Sharon. "And then to have the doctors not believe me made the whole process that much harder."

Eventually, an obstetrician-gynecologist performed an ultrasound, found a large cyst growing outside her uterus, and diagnosed Sharon with endometriosis. The condition develops when the tissue that normally lines the inside of the uterus (the endometrium) grows outside of the uterus, causing intense pain, particularly during menstrual periods. Endometriosis is often found in women who have fibromyalgia.

After Sharon's cyst was removed and her endometriosis was treated with hormonal medication, the pain lessened. She graduated with a degree in public relations, got a job in that field, and managed to function—even ride her bike, go to the gym, and rollerblade regularly. But the pain was always there. "Just before I turned twenty-four, I got severe bronchitis in the winter and it just wouldn't improve; it lasted for weeks and weeks. Around the same time, I started to have more pain in my body. I remember being at work and looking under my shirt jacket for bruises. It hurt so badly, I thought there had to be a bruise or mark," says Sharon.

There was no visible mark. But Sharon began to see her problem more clearly when she sought relief one day by going to get a massage, and the massage therapist suggested she could have fibromyalgia. At the time Sharon didn't even know what that was, but she investigated and soon found a rheumatologist. At that appointment, for the first time, she was properly diagnosed with fibromyalgia. The autoimmune disorder, characterized by widespread musculoskeletal pain along with fatigue and mood issues, had likely been simmering for years, underlying all of Sharon's pain without her knowing it.

Unfortunately, the diagnosis did not usher in a new phase of relief. Instead, the rheumatologist told Sharon she'd have to learn to live with fibromyalgia without so much as a conversation. "He told me to stop exercising and to rest, and then he literally threw a brochure at me from the Arthritis Foundation, and gave me a prescription for antidepressants, and left the room," says Sharon. "That was my whole 'welcome to fibro' talk."

Without any real explanation of the disease or support for her treatment, Sharon didn't understand the rationale for the antidepressants, so she didn't take them. But she did follow the doctor's recommendation to stop exercising. Within a month, she was bedridden. "I couldn't sleep and I couldn't walk," she says. "I couldn't even walk from the bedroom to the bathroom without lying down for a nap, that's how fatigued I was." Her symptoms had spiraled into a full-blown fibromyalgia flare.

Sharon had to take a three-month leave from her job. She had no idea what had happened to her. Little did she know that the exercise she'd been doing all along had actually been helping her body stay strong, or that the antidepressants she'd been prescribed would have helped her sleep. As it happened, however, Sharon's mom, looking for some way to help her daughter, had contacted the Arthritis Foundation—one of the few resources for rheumatologic diseases available to them at the time—and learned of a water aerobics class being offered locally, geared to people with arthritis. The buoyancy of the water enabled people in pain to exercise with less pressure on their joints.

Sharon almost didn't make it to the class. "The class was in the pool of a hotel and I had to walk through the whole lobby to get to the locker room, which was more than I could handle at the time. I was just in so much pain, I sat in the hotel crying," remembers Sharon about that first day at the aerobics class. "When I finally got to the pool and the instructor asked me what was wrong, I told her about my pain, and she told me that she had fibro, too." Yet the instructor wasn't doubled over crying, she noted. She was bouncing and gliding around the pool, like a ray of hope. "That was a life changing moment," remembers Sharon. "She literally helped me get back on my feet again and showed me that I could have a life, even with fibromyalgia."

After that glimpse of a possible future, Sharon made recovery her full-time job. She went to either physical therapy or water aerobics at least four days a week—even though, on the days she participated in one of those activities, it was all she could manage to do. The rest of the day she had to lie in bed. Sharon, still in her mid-twenties, felt as if she was living the life of someone decades older, which was depressing and terrifying. But she pushed through. "It was out of survival," she says. "I knew I needed to continue and to find something that I was interested in or that brought me joy, or I wouldn't be able to go on."

Sharon went to see a different rheumatologist who worked with her to find appropriate medications. First, she tried muscle relaxants, but they made her hallucinate and sleepwalk, so she discontinued those. Eventually an antidepressant improved her sleep. Still, she was scared and felt alone in her struggle, so she tried going to a support group organized by the Arthritis Foundation. But she couldn't relate to the people there: "I was the youngest person in the room by far, and most of the people there had walkers and wheelchairs. I'd leave feeling more depressed than when I came."

Sharon went searching for help across the country. She attended a scientific meeting in Oregon where researchers from all over the world talked about their work in fibromyalgia. "When I found people who really understood the disease, that's when I finally started to apply their teachings to my care." She then trained to become a fibromyalgia leader through the Arthritis Foundation, doing what she could to fill the void of information that existed for fibromyalgia patients at the time. "I was so mad about how the doctors had dismissed my symptoms for all those years, and I wanted to do something to educate and support others," she says.

In 1997, Sharon founded the St. John Hospital Fibromyalgia Support and Education Group, which, by 2003, grew into the Fibromyalgia Association of Michigan, in Warren, where she holds monthly meetings. At her very first meeting, seventy people affected by fibromyalgia showed up. "People came up to me in tears thanking me for starting the group," Sharon says. At that time, there were just a couple of books on fibromyalgia, and the internet was just developing. People were desperate for this information."

Today, as a certified lifestyle medicine health and wellness coach, Sharon continues to run the fibromyalgia group as founder and president. Married with two teenage children, she has a busy life and is keeping her fibro under control. She takes an antidepressant to help her sleep, is mindful of what she eats, and exercises six days a week. "It's not a choice. It's like brushing my teeth," she says. "I have to do it." She has learned—through years of trial and error—to treat her fibromyalgia with a multidisciplinary approach combining medication, physical therapy, occupational therapy, psychological interventions, exercise, and nutrition.

Looking back on her childhood, Sharon can't help imagining what might have been if her doctors had only understood the cause of her pain and taken it seriously. If her "growing pains" had been accurately diagnosed as juvenile-onset fibromyalgia and she'd been able to get appropriate treatment when she was a child, her illness might not have progressed so far. "If someone had explained to me what to do to treat my fibro initially, I really think that I wouldn't have wound up the way I did," says Sharon. But her experience inspires her all the more to help others. "We're still seeing that it takes an average of five years to get a diagnosis of fibromyalgia, and if we could get those diagnoses sooner, the levels of disability would be lower," she says. "I really want people to get off to a better start."

Reluctantly Labeled

Though researchers' understanding of juvenile-onset fibromyalgia has grown immensely in the more than thirty years since Sharon was a child, much remains to be discovered about its origins, progression, and treatment. There is even still debate among clinicians about whether or not children should be labeled as having fibromyalgia. "Fibromyalgia is very well recognized in adults, but it hasn't been as well recognized in children, and that's not because the disease isn't seen in pediatric clinics," says Susmita Kashikar-Zuck, professor of pediatrics and clinical anesthesiology at Cincinnati Children's Hospital Medical Center, and director of behavioral medicine and clinical psychology research there. "Chronic, widespread musculoskeletal pain is a fairly common complaint in specialized pain centers and in rheumatology clinics, and also in some other specialties," she adds, "but over the years, physicians have been reluctant to assign the classification of fibromyalgia to children because not a lot was known about it, or physicians thought maybe children would grow out of it, or they felt that maybe the diagnostic label involved some type of stigma."

Dr. Kashikar-Zuck has done extensive work to raise awareness about fibromyalgia in children because she knows that this historical hesitance to recognize it has meant that families typically go from doctor to doctor searching for answers without getting properly diagnosed or treated for months or years. "With fibromyalgia, patients complain of pain," she explains, "but there is typically no obvious sign of inflammation or any blood test or biomarker that doctors can identify." A child with fibromyalgia may have various pains in addition to musculoskeletal pain—ranging from headaches to stomachaches—and often sees a pediatrician, a neurologist, or gastroenterologist before eventually being referred to a pain clinic or a rheumatologist. "Out of all types of pain conditions," she notes, "fibromyalgia is particularly complex and it is one of the most disabling."

Early in her career, Dr. Kashikar-Zuck felt compelled to focus on juvenile-onset fibromyalgia because she saw it as an "orphan diagnosis." Children with the disease (typically adolescent girls) were dismissed by doctors, and their excruciating pain was left undertreated. The need for more research in the field was evident, so when she began to specialize in the late 1990s she rose to the challenge.

Through research like Dr. Kashikar-Zuck's, along with the work of patient advocates like Sharon, we now know that juvenile-onset fibromyalgia is very real: there are underlying physiological differences between people with fibromyalgia and people without the condition. We also know that the disease tends to follow children into adulthood.[12] But the research is making a positive difference. "There has been huge progress in the last twenty years," says Dr. Kashikar-Zuck. As doctors investigate the disease, they are constantly improving treatment protocols.

What Causes Juvenile-Onset Fibromyalgia?

There isn't a great deal of research indicating what might trigger fibromyalgia in children, but Dr. Kashikar-Zuck has seen across her decades of study that symptoms often start with an infection—like a severe flu or stomach bug—that affects the immune system. For instance, in Sharon, her fibromyalgia seemed to develop in full force after an intense bout of bronchitis. In these cases, the immune system response goes awry and alters how the nervous system functions. That said, fibromyalgia can also start stealthily with pain in one part of the body that then insidiously spreads and is accompanied by fatigue and sleep problems. But because most research in fibromyalgia has been conducted with adults who've typically had the condition for decades, we still know very little about the biology and causes of the condition in children.

Also, like CRPS, the causes of juvenile fibromyalgia are complex. Scientists believe the disease is influenced by peripheral and central nervous system factors, gene expression changes, and immune factors, but the research is still in its infancy. As Dr. Kashikar-Zuck puts it, "It's taken the field of pain research a long time to recognize that chronic pain in children is a problem that we need to pay attention to—and that children won't necessarily just grow out of it. So we're just now getting to drill down a little deeper into why this is happening at such an early age. Why is it happening more in girls than in boys? What are some of the hormonal influences, for example? Those studies are all just starting."

Managing Fibromyalgia and the Fear That Accompanies It

Adolescents dealing with fibromyalgia—a disease that is invisible yet all-encompassing—often feel anxious, depressed, and alone. When the pain of the illness keeps them from participating in school or other normal teenage activities (as it often does), they feel even more isolated and despondent. But there is reason to be hopeful. Research has shown that a combination of cognitive behavioral therapy, exercise, physical therapy, and medication can lessen both pain and depression, and help kids return to the activities of their daily lives.[13]

As with CRPS, though, for many children with fibromyalgia, the *fear* of pain remains crippling—both emotionally and physically. "I've noticed that even when adolescents start to get back to some of their social and academic activities, they are still not physically active at all, because exercise was something that was very, very scary for them," says Dr. Kashikar-Zuck. "And even after seeing significant improvement in their pain levels, every time they'd start to move or do something vigorous, they would complain that their body would hurt more."

To address the fear of movement and the pain it seemed to cause, Dr. Kashikar-Zuck decided to study this phenomenon. She discovered that children with fibromyalgia actually learn to move in maladaptive ways after years of compromised physical activity. Her research reveals what happens when children feel intense pain each time they walk, run, or simply get out of bed: over a period of time, they learn ways to protect themselves. To prevent pain, they alter the biomechanics of how they get around in the world, and end up creating other problems. "If you watch a young person who has musculoskeletal pain for a long time, you can actually see that their gait, their posture, their balance, and their confidence in movement really changes because they're guarding, and they're trying not to hurt themselves," explains Dr. Kashikar-Zuck. "And unfortunately, the way you move your body has a lot to do with injury and pain." Fear and avoidance of healthy movement therefore perpetuates disabling movement patterns that increase susceptibility to pain.[14]

"So you've got doctors saying, 'Well, you really need to get into physical therapy. You need to do regular exercise,'" Dr. Kashikar-Zuck notes. "But how do you tell a teenager to exercise, when they associate exercise with increasing pain?" An answer to that, she thought, could be found in sports medicine, where specialists constantly help athletes with injury prevention. "When I looked at what they were doing, a lot of it made sense to me in terms of its application for chronic musculoskeletal pain. Because what the sports medicine doctors and coaches do is teach their athletes how to move their bodies, essentially, without hurting or injuring themselves, so that they can be at peak performance. And imagine, if you're moving your body with altered biomechanics, it doesn't matter how much you exercise, because as soon as you start to move your body, you're moving it in a way that's injury prone, and it's going to hurt."

This simple yet revelatory idea led Dr. Kashikar-Zuck to take a step back before simply prescribing exercise to children with fibromyalgia. Instead of telling the kids to "start small" and start walking on a treadmill for five minutes a day, she realized she would need to help them retrain their bodies to move first. Just as the nervous system needs retraining during recovery, so does the musculoskeletal system.

Dr. Kashikar-Zuck has since started a neuromuscular training program called FIT Teens (the acronym stands for Fibromyalgia Integrative Training). Still in the pilot stage, the ongoing study involves seven locations across the United States and Canada. Using computers to perform sophisticated biomechanics analysis in a 3D-motion lab ("a kind of Pixar technology," says Dr. Kashikar-Zuck), researchers put retro-reflective markers on teenagers' joints, and track their movements before they begin any treatment. "There are thirty-six different markers, and ten cameras all around, and we have them do different tasks like walking, and jumping, and balancing while taking a full 3D-motion-capture analysis," she explains.[15]

Kids in the FIT Teens treatment program come in twice a week for eight weeks to practice specialized exercises that help them move safely while improving their strength, posture, and balance. "They also learn skills to cope with pain and fear of movement," adds Dr. Kashikar-Zuck. After the completion of the program, the teenagers' biomechanics are measured again with the 3D-motion-capture system to see how they've progressed.

The results so far are very promising, and the researchers see measurable improvements in the kids' movement patterns and posture after completing the program. "They're moving with greater force and strength, but moving in a correct manner," reports Dr. Kashikar-Zuck, "so that they're not putting uneven force on different joints in their body in an effort to prevent pain flares from happening."

The program has other important benefits, too. It teaches kids how to differentiate between fibromyalgia pain and normal, exercise-induced muscle soreness. And the kids have the opportunity to work in groups with other teens. In many cases, this is the first time they have ever met another teenager suffering with chronic pain. The kids learn from each other (in addition to the trainers) and support each other, which helps them stay motivated and engaged.[16]

Dr. Kashikar-Zuck's next objective is to evaluate whether these treatments are able to alter neuropathways. She is hoping to begin a study that uses neuroimaging before and after treatment to see if there are changes to the central nervous system and pain network. "Because we've seen changes in strength, we've seen changes in emotional aspects, and the way the whole brain is perceiving pain," she explains, "our hypothesis is that this nonpharmacologic treatment is actually going to have a biological effect."

Can Medication Help Treat Juvenile-Onset Fibromyalgia?

Currently, there are no medications for juvenile-onset fibromyalgia that have been approved by the US Food and Drug Administration specifically for children. There are three medications that have been approved for adults with fibromyalgia. Pregabalin, the generic version of Lyrica, is used to treat nerve pain and seizures. Duloxetine is in a class of antidepressants called selective serotonin and norepinephrine reuptake inhibitors—known as SSNRIs—and can be used to treat anxiety, neuropathy, and chronic muscle or bone pain. Milnacipran is in a class of antidepressants called serotonin-norepinephrine reuptake inhibitors—known as SNRIs—and is used to treat fibromyalgia pain. While studies are underway to test these medications in children with fibromyalgia, the results are not yet in.

Physicians do sometimes prescribe these medications to children under close supervision, but there are significant downsides. For example, many of these medications tend to increase drowsiness, which interferes with school, and some of these drugs may increase the risk of suicidal ideation. As a result, both doctors and parents are very careful about trying these medications in children. Most often kids are prescribed low-doses of three types of medication, sometimes in combination, to help with mood and sleep difficulties: amitriptyline, an antidepressant that treats anxiety, depression, and pain; cyclobenzaprine, a muscle relaxant; and antidepressants such as SNRIs or SSRIs (selective serotonin reuptake inhibitors). In some children, oral contraceptives can also help quell severe menstrual cramps. Non-steroidal anti-inflammatory drugs (NSAIDs) and opioids are typically ineffective in alleviating fibromyalgia symptoms.

Juvenile-Onset Fibromyalgia and Hope for the Future

As things stand today, about 50 percent of teenagers with fibromyalgia grow into adults who have full-blown fibromyalgia, and almost all teenagers with fibromyalgia continue to experience at least one of the cardinal symptoms of the disease in adulthood: widespread pain, sleep disturbances, and fatigue.[17] But there is reason to believe we can change these outcomes. Researchers and physicians are beginning to focus much more on treating this condition in childhood. "I think people are realizing that if you can catch these pain syndromes early, and treat them effectively, you can avoid the huge problems that accompany chronic pain in adulthood," says Dr. Kashikar-Zuck. Children's nervous systems are still developing and are very plastic—and are not nearly as hardwired as adults' systems are, so there is the potential to have a big impact on pain pathways in childhood. In the case of juvenile fibromyalgia, early interventions such as cognitive behavioral therapy and neuromuscular training may also give adolescents the possibility of a future with much less pain. "We may not be able to make the pain get to zero," Dr. Kashikar-Zuck allows, "but we can minimize it to the extent that children can basically continue their daily activities, go to college, have relationships, have children, and lead relatively normal lives."

This hope is what keeps Dr. Kashikar-Zuck and other pediatric pain researchers going. "We see kids get better, and we see their families get back on track," she says. "I have a lot of optimism for where we're going."

Chapter 10

More than Just Medication

Multidisciplinary treatments for
lessening children's suffering

There are few things more heart-wrenching for parents than seeing their child in pain, especially when they see no clear path toward relief. As we've discussed, chronic pain in children is complex, and the misconceptions about how to handle it are many. Although effective interdisciplinary treatments exist, not enough people know about these strategies and they're not easily accessible to all who need them. More often than not, families struggle for months or years while navigating a complicated medical system. Kids with chronic pain often see a slew of clinicians in a variety of specialties before they find their way to a comprehensive pediatric pain center— if they ever do. And research shows that the longer children have to wait to find appropriate care, the more anxiety and frustration they tend to feel.[1]

Fortunately, pediatric pain centers are growing in number across the country and internationally. There are now approximately eighty-three such centers worldwide, including about fifty pediatric pain centers in North America.[2] They are typically staffed by a combination of physicians, psychologists (like Anna), and physical therapists working together to help manage children's pain. Kids may go to pain programs for inpatient care, for intensive outpatient care, or for periodic visits, depending on their needs. While there are not yet enough pediatric pain centers to meet the demand of the estimated three million to five million children in the United States who experience chronic pain, the dedicated professionals who work in these programs do their best to let pediatric medical providers know these programs exist, and how they can reduce kids' suffering, improve their mood, get them back to school, and help them live their full lives.[3] The more that pediatric providers refer families to these programs, the more children will benefit.

Further, in recent years, clinicians have been making concerted efforts to expand their offerings by making some pain treatments available online or via telemedicine, a strategy that became especially critical when the Covid-19 pandemic made many in-person visits impossible. The results of these online treatments are promising. One recent study led by pediatric psychologist Lynn Walker focused on children with functional abdominal pain and revealed that kids' symptoms can be lessened with either pain education or cognitive behavioral therapy (CBT) delivered via the internet. Further, while the more expensive of these two options—the online therapy, involving personal interactions with a health coach—was more effective for the subgroup of children classified as "high pain dysfunctional," kids in the two other subgroups (those experiencing high pain but with greater adaptive responses, and those experiencing lower pain) benefited equally from the online pain education.[4] "The point being, parents who don't have access or financial resources for CBT should not despair—other options may be equally beneficial," says Dr. Walker. Whether families find their way to pain centers in person or use online services remotely, the help can be life-changing.

Fiona's Story: Finding the Right Care

"Going to the pain clinic at Boston Children's Hospital was the best thing that happened to us," says Fiona, from Maine, who was referred to the center when she was thirteen. At that point she had suffered three years of chronic joint pain and intense headaches, caused by a combination of Lyme disease and a series of concussions, and had seen her pediatrician, an osteopathic doctor, a neurologist, a Lyme disease specialist, and an occupational therapist. None of those practitioners had been able to prescribe an approach or medication that helped her. Between her fifth- and eighth-grade years, Fiona endured varying levels of pain which often kept her out of school.

When Fiona arrived at Boston Children's as an eighth-grader, she'd missed school and soccer practice for more than a month and, because of her extreme sensitivity to light, sound, and electronic screens, she had spent the majority of that time in bed in the dark by herself. "Emotionally, I was pretty depressed because I couldn't be in school and I did love being in school, and I couldn't spend any time with my friends," remembers Fiona. "It was very lonely, and I really didn't have a good idea of what was going on." But her outlook and her outcome eventually changed after she began working with a Boston Children's pediatric pain team made up of clinicians who knew how to treat her pain and could teach her how to manage it.

How Interdisciplinary Pain Management Works

Interdisciplinary pain management, incorporating a variety of medical and psychological specialties, has been mentioned in prior chapters. What does it actually look like in practice? In the pediatric pain management clinic at Oregon Health and Science University, where Anna works, the clinical team often explains to families that having chronic pain is like having four flat tires, and to get kids moving again, they need to figure out how to fill each of them. Depending on the child, the best way to fill one tire might be with medication, while a second might call for cognitive behavioral therapy, a third for physical therapy or other type of movement, and a fourth for yet a different non-medication approach, such as acupuncture, nutrition changes, returning to social activities with friends, or adjusting the child's sleep schedule. Each child's treatment is different and multifaceted, which is why having a team of pain-treatment professionals tends to be most effective.

Most formal pediatric pain programs include at least three core disciplines, so that children work with a physical therapist, a pain psychologist, and a physician (usually a pediatric anesthesiologist, rehabilitation physician, or pediatrician who has gained advanced training or experience in pain management). Often, programs also include nurse practitioners or occupational therapists, and sometimes they offer more services such as acupuncture, biofeedback, massage, nutritional guidance, and parent support groups.

Just as important as the variety of practitioners on these teams is the fact that they share a philosophy and treatment approach. The teams are dedicated first and foremost to improving functioning for kids whose lives have been derailed by pain. As Fiona's story illustrates, by the time most families get to a pain treatment center, the kids have typically missed many days of school, fallen behind academically, had to quit sports teams. Some have drifted apart from friends and are dealing with anxiety or depression. The first goal, which surprises many families, is not to relieve all pain immediately—

because in many cases, that is not feasible. Instead, the primary goal is to get kids functioning again, and to teach them how to return to their lives while managing the pain. Once kids can do that, pain relief often follows.[5]

Psychoeducation Is Vital

One of the core components of pediatric pain programs is teaching both the children and their parents about pain. Research shows that kids (and adults) experience improvement in their functioning and symptoms after simply learning more about how pain works in the body and brain, how pain can become chronic, and why gradually returning to activity can help turn down the dial on a hypersensitive nervous system and reduce pain over time.[6] Indeed, this is territory we covered in Chapter 1.

Fiona's education began when she started meeting weekly with her pediatric pain psychologist at Boston Children's, Rachael Coakley, who is also an associate professor at Harvard Medical School and director of clinical innovation and outreach in pain medicine. "I didn't know a whole lot about chronic pain," says Fiona. "Rachael was able to teach me ways to handle my pain, and work through it in a way that didn't involve medication—to help myself."

Dr. Coakley also validated that Fiona's pain was real, and that even though psychological problems weren't the cause of her pain, there were psychological tools she could use to alleviate it. "We help families understand that there are really effective, evidence-based psychological strategies to treat chronic pain in the long-term," says Dr. Coakley. "The strategies are not a Band-Aid for pain, or a temporary fix. They are not something to do until your medication kicks in. They are fantastic interventions that can truly help to reduce pain and improve function in a wide variety of conditions, and they are often overlooked outside of pain centers."

These psychological strategies often include evidence-based treatments of three kinds: cognitive behavioral therapy to address anxiety and insomnia; physiological self-regulation therapies such as self-hypnosis, guided imagery, mindfulness-based stress reduction, and biofeedback (all of which train the brain to respond to the body's physiological functions); and parent coaching. In a number of studies, such psychological treatments alone have been shown to improve children's chronic pain, particularly when parents are involved in delivering them.[7] But at an interdisciplinary pain clinic, such strategies are typically combined with physical therapy, occupational therapy, and medication, as needed. For each family a comprehensive plan is devised, specific to their case.[8]

A Tailored Pain Plan

Part of the beauty of having a whole pain team supporting a family is that treatment components can be delivered by different professionals on the team at different times, depending on what works best for the child and parents. For instance, a teenage boy with chronic back pain and sleep problems might receive cognitive behavioral therapy from a pain psychologist, and he may work with a physical therapist on movement to reduce fear of pain. The team nurse practitioner might connect with the family over the phone to adjust the timing of medication doses to improve sleep, and to help the family find a yoga class in their community or a mindfulness class at school. The family might also check in with the pediatric anesthesiologist if medications have troublesome side effects or if other issues arise.

Throughout treatment, the team can continue to lay out different options in consultation with the parents and child and refine the customized plan. When circumstances change and the plan needs adjusting, the team can continue to advise.

There are also programs that combine specific aspects of psychological therapies with specific aspects of physical therapy to target subgroups of children with chronic pain. For instance, Laura Simons, a pediatric pain psychologist and associate professor at Stanford University, has developed a program called "GET Living" that is aimed at treating kids with high levels of pain-related fear. The program (available as part of a clinical trial at the time of this writing) incorporates gradual behavioral exposure to feared movements with physical therapy.[9]

Not only do such pain programs work, but there is also emerging evidence that they are cost-effective for the patients and for the medical system. Researchers have found that when children are treated through an interdisciplinary chronic pain clinic, patient care expenses come down drastically.[10] Fewer emergency room visits, fewer expensive specialty consultations, and fewer overall visits to the doctor add up to lower costs.

Setting Expectations about Pharmaceuticals, Including Opioids

What should parents know about pharmaceuticals if they are just beginning to seek treatment for a child's pain? First, it's important to keep in mind that there is usually no magic pill that can alleviate chronic pain. As appealing as a quick fix would be, medications are best implemented as part of a multifaceted plan for addressing chronic pain.[11] Second, be aware that the medications that often work to treat *acute* pain in kids are less effective for treating chronic pain. (Remember, acute pain and chronic pain often don't respond to the same modalities.) The medications typically used for acute pain include over-the-counter analgesics (such as Tylenol, a brand of acetaminophen), non-steroidal anti-inflammatory medications (such as Advil, a brand of ibuprofen), and prescription opioids (also called narcotics), which attach to receptors in the central nervous system and brain and block pain signals.

A note about opioids: these controversial prescription drugs do have an important place in managing children's acute pain in certain situations, as we discussed in Chapter 5. For example, opioids can be effective and necessary in quelling a child's post-surgical pain. They can mitigate pain flares in kids with diseases where pain stimulation is known to be part of the disease (such as cancer and sickle cell anemia).[12] But opioids are not generally recommended for treating primary pain disorders (like headaches or stomachaches) in kids. Why? For starters, opioids are not highly effective in these instances. Further, opioids carry serious side effects—including nausea, constipation, breathing issues, and cognitive impairment—which don't tend to outweigh their benefits in the case of chronic pain. In fact, many adults with chronic pain have found opioids to be intolerable.[13] Of course, opioids also carry the severe risk of misuse, addiction, and life-threatening overdose if they are used without the supervision of a knowledgeable physician.[14]

While the dangers of misuse and addiction have been highly publicized, there are ways to mitigate the risks if your child requires opioids.[15] Jennifer Rabbitts, associate professor of pain medicine at the University of Washington School of Medicine and attending anesthesiologist at the Seattle Children's Hospital, stresses that families must work with their doctors to establish expectations about how long the child may need to take opioids, to be prepared to wean off of them, and to learn how to dispose of them. It is vital, when the treatment is finished, that remaining doses don't get misused either recreationally or accidentally (if, for instance, a young child in the home finds the pills). "Unfortunately, there are times when a child is prescribed oxycodone—without having tried nonopioid analgesics first—and they're given no instructions on how often to take them, how to taper down, and what to do with the leftover pills," says Dr. Rabbitts. This can be especially problematic if the child has risk factors for opioid misuse (for instance, a personal history of opioid addiction).

The message, then, is to be judicious about using opioids and to follow these guidelines:

- Do not share opioid medications with any other family members.
- Monitor your child's usage carefully.
- Secure the pills so that they are inaccessible to children of all ages.
- Check in with the prescribing doctor about any side effects that arise.
- Ask the prescribing doctor when and how to wean off the medication if your child uses it for more than a few days.
- Do not keep leftover pills for later use.
- Follow instructions on the label or from your doctor or pharmacist about how to discard unused pills. (Depending on the drug, you may be instructed not to flush the pills but rather to instead mix them with coffee grounds, dirt, or cat litter and put them in the trash.)

Managing Medications for Chronic Pain

The pharmaceuticals that physicians do tend to prescribe to help children manage common chronic pain conditions include antidepressants (such as Cymbalta, a brand of duloxetine), anti-seizure medications (such as Neurontin, a brand of gabapentin), and nerve pain medications (such as Lyrica, a brand of pregabalin). All of these are thought to target an oversensitive nervous system, albeit in different ways. Doctors may also prescribe children muscle relaxants (such as Valium, a brand of diazepam) or topical anti-inflammatory creams or patches for use on a short-term basis (such as lidocaine). There are numerous other pharmaceuticals to consider—this list is far from exhaustive—and all medications carry the risk of side effects. Anyone seeking medication for their child's chronic pain should be aware that it often takes trial and error, under the care of a prescribing healthcare provider, to arrive at the prescription with the greatest benefit and least downside.

Also, as discussed in Chapter 9, remember that many of the medications used to treat chronic pain have not been expressly approved by the US Food and Drug Administration for use with children. Because the clinical trials required for drug approvals rarely include children, pediatric physicians are charged with using their best judgment when making decisions about these medications. In the best-case scenario, the doctor and parents work closely together—along with the rest of a child's pain management team—to review medication options, discuss each medication's pros and cons, and carefully monitor the child throughout treatment.

In some cases, a child's pain team may also refer families to a naturopath or registered dietician who might incorporate nutritional supplements, probiotics, herbs, aromatherapy, or cannabidiol (often abbreviated to CBD, a chemical compound from the cannabis plant that does not have a psychogenic effect). While there is less research on the effects of these options in children, ideally, the pain team would evaluate the benefits and risks of any modality as part of a child's overall care.

Maddy's Story: The Value of Being Heard

While every pain program is different, a component they all tend to share is a staff committed to truly listening to the families they see. Typically, by the time patients find their way to a pediatric pain clinic, they've exhausted almost every other option. The children have usually been told more than once that they are either making up the pain or that there is nothing that can be done for them. At a pain clinic, families should always expect to be heard.

That's what happened to Maddy and her family, who live in Ottawa, Canada. Maddy had an unusual, and extremely painful, problem with her shoulder. Beginning when she was fourteen years old, the round part of her upper arm bone repeatedly became dislocated from its socket. The family would end up in the emergency department three times a week to get it put back in place, recalls Joan, Maddy's mother, who notes that the family's pediatrician couldn't offer specialized care. "It went on for months like this, and it got to the point where we'd arrive at the hospital, and the doctors would shame us for being there," Joan says. "Once they saw we were repeat customers at the emergency department, and that we were bringing her in for the same problem, they would throw up their hands and tell us it wasn't an emergency, and that it was all in her head."

But the problem persisted and the pain only got worse. In fact, it spread—to her other shoulder, to her neck, to most of her joints, and finally throughout her body. She began having stomachaches, headaches, breathing difficulties, and fevers. The previously easy-going teenager was forced to stop attending school and spent all her time in bed.

The orthopedic surgeons Maddy saw offered no solutions, and the family became desperate. "We couldn't understand why no one would help her," says Joan. After about six months, during one emergency room visit, the doctor there decided to perform an emergency surgery on Maddy's shoulder, but that led to even more excruciating pain. "The day she came home from surgery, her pain was unbearable. We'd never seen anything like it. It was terrifying. We were beside ourselves. We had to take her back to the hospital," remembers Joan. "She was screaming in agony, thrashing, fevered, and sweaty, and they wound up admitting her for about a week but there was still a lot of skepticism about her pain."

After that horrific episode, the family was referred to the Hospital for Sick Children (SickKids) in Toronto where the doctors diagnosed the problem: Maddy had Ehlers-Danlos Syndrome, a genetic disorder that weakens the body's connective tissues and causes overly flexible joints, along with thin, fragile skin. It is known to lead to extreme musculoskeletal pain. Some variants of the syndrome can also weaken blood vessels and organs, causing further complications.

Getting the diagnosis was key to finding a solution, but it wasn't until Maddy and her parents went to the Mayo Clinic in Rochester, Minnesota, that she began to find relief. Participating in an intensive three-week outpatient program there focused on pediatric pain rehabilitation, she was taught how to function despite her disease. The family had a medical team helping them assess pharmaceutical options and providing psychological help, physical therapy, occupational therapy, biofeedback, recreational therapy, and parent coaching. They learned about the importance of sleep, finding spiritual connections, and striking a balance among school, family, social life, hobbies, and physical activity. "We learned that the pain will always be there but, the more you figure out how to live a balanced life, the less intense the pain will be, and the fewer bad days you'll have," says Joan. "Also, the community of support the program offered to families and children was tremendous. Having other people who understood the experience of living with chronic pain was so helpful."

Maddy, now twenty-one years old, is pursuing an undergraduate degree in child development and plans to become a teacher. Joan credits the pediatric pain program with instilling in Maddy how to live her life without letting the disease take center stage. "She prioritizes nutrition and exercise, as well as time with family and friends and school," says Joan. "The program also helped her to regain access to the part of herself that experiences gratitude every day for life's simple pleasures. I want to be more like my daughter when I grow up!"

A Parent's Supporting Role

One aspect of a pain program that is especially central to its success is how it helps parents understand their role in supporting their child. For many parents, this may take some retraining. In the majority of families who've been saddled with chronic pain, for example, the parents often focus all of their energies on trying to ease their child's discomfort. They may hasten to wait on their child, let her stay home from school and watch favorite TV shows, and let her off the hook for homework, chores, or other obligations. These are well-intentioned and natural tendencies for loving parents who feel there is little else they can do to help. Who wouldn't want to give their struggling child a little respite? The problem with being overly solicitous, though, is that it can encourage a child to dwell on the pain, remain immobilized, and withdraw from normal life—making a bad situation worse. As we've highlighted, when parents show high levels of distress and are overly protective of their child in pain, this can cause the child's functioning to deteriorate.[16]

Studies show that when parents consistently attend to their child's pain (for instance, by repeatedly asking "Are you ok?" or "Does that hurt a lot?" or "How is your pain today?"), children tend to complain of more pain. Conversely, when parents distract from the pain—maybe by playing a board game or talking about weekend plans—children experience less discomfort.[17] To be clear, this does not mean that parents should discount their child's pain. Rather, as we've discussed, one of the most helpful things a parent can do for a child in pain is build up the child's self-confidence and signal that the child has the ability to get through the obstacle.

Psychologists at pediatric pain programs, therefore, work with parents to help them manage their own distress and minimize their own catastrophizing, as well as teach them how to support their children's learning and use of new tools to regain functioning. This seems to work well for both the parents and the kids. For instance, Joan notes that a strength of the Mayo Clinic program was that it integrated the families, offering them emotional support and providing education about when and how to be there for their children.

Fiona, at Boston Children's, also noticed that her parents were better able to support her after spending time with the pain team. "My parents used to ask me every five minutes how I was feeling, and they learned to stop doing that, which gave me the space to approach them when I needed," she says. "We also learned how to communicate with each other about my pain in a productive way so they could understand what I was feeling, and trust me in what I said I could and couldn't do. So, I would be able to explain to them that I'm feeling okay enough to wash the dishes tonight but I don't know if I can spend the whole day at school tomorrow."

Figuring out when to stand back and when to push your child with a chronic pain condition is difficult. There is no rule book on how to do it. "We realize that parents are not born with the parenting skills of knowing what to do with a child in chronic pain," says Susmita Kashikar-Zuck, a professor of pediatrics and clinical anesthesiology at Cincinnati Children's Hospital Medical Center who researches fibromyalgia in children. "And you still need to have ground rules, and you still need to have the family functioning in a normative way so that the whole family dynamic doesn't get completely thrown off-kilter by having a child who is in pain all the time, which can very easily happen." Clinicians usually find that the treatment process works best when parents serve as a positive support system. "Let us be the bad guys," Dr. Kashikar-Zuck advises: "let us do this training part, and then you just be the good coach and the cheerleader."

Dr. Coakley agrees that educating parents is essential. "There is so much evidence showing that, across all interventions for kids with pain, when you support parents, the kids get better," she says. "I think empowering parents through teaching and evidence-based parent training is a critical component of all pediatric pain care."

Innovations in Treatment: Getting Effective
Pain Management to Everyone

In the cases of both Fiona and Maddy, the family had to travel to another state to receive treatment at a specialized pediatric pain clinic. This is not uncommon, because many states don't have one. But not everyone can get to a clinic far away from their home. What's more, many families face other obstacles such as financial constraints, health insurance barriers, difficulties taking time off from work to support the child's treatment, and competing demands of other family needs. Enrolling in a pediatric pain clinic can be a substantial commitment of time and resources, and beyond that, the treatment also typically requires adherence to therapies that must be incorporated into a child's daily routine. For any number of reasons, going to a specialized clinic might not be possible.[18] In these cases, families may be able to put together their own version of a multidisciplinary pain management team within their community; the process starts with asking a pediatrician for referrals to local practitioners such as pediatric psychologists and physical therapists, and for help in coordinating the care. There is also another alternative: increasingly, pain researchers are developing ways to offer pain care remotely, so kids can access it no matter where they are.

One such initiative is called Web-Based Management of Adolescent Pain (WebMAP), which is an online intervention for children with chronic pain and their parents. WebMAP is currently downloadable as a smart phone application and offers a six-week, virtual program of cognitive behavioral therapy. Families using it learn about chronic pain and are trained on tools that can help them improve mood, sleep, relaxation, and function—all from their home. As well as teaching strategies such as mindfulness and deep breathing, the program enables kids to set personal goals for increasing their physical activity and then track their progress. Research has found WebMAP to be effective in reducing pain and improving function.[19]

WebMAP was conceived in 2005 by Tonya Palermo, when she was the only psychologist in the pediatric pain management clinic at Doernbecher Children's Hospital in Portland, Oregon (where Anna now works). In fact, Dr. Palermo was the only pediatric psychologist specializing in pain in the entire state of Oregon at the time, and she realized that she alone couldn't possibly see all the children in the area who needed help. Demand for her services was so high that patients often had to wait months for an appointment, and sometimes she would learn that a family had driven up to six hours (one way!) to have that one-hour session.

Frustration fuels innovation. "After seeing patients who had traveled from four to six hours for their visits, it became very clear that the only way to ensure that children and families could receive evidence-based psychological treatment for chronic pain was to administer treatment to them online," says Dr. Palermo. In 2006 Anna began her postdoctoral fellowship at Doernbecher Children's Hospital, with Dr. Palermo as her supervisor, and helped develop and test the new program for its first pilot study.[20] Anna and Dr. Palermo saw how useful it was for families to be able to receive pain management care without having to take long, stressful drives to access it.

Now a professor of anesthesia and pain medicine at Seattle Children's Hospital in Washington, Dr. Palermo has continued to refine and improve WebMAP. During the Covid-19 pandemic, the program became even more necessary. "At the beginning of the pandemic we developed a guide on how to integrate the app into telehealth visits, during a time when in-person healthcare visits largely halted," says Dr. Palermo.

While WebMAP was one of the first online interventions for pediatric pain, several additional programs have since been developed
that offer help for managing pediatric pain remotely.[21] Looking to
the horizon, a growing number of virtual reality programs in development also show promise. These VR systems, using headsets to provide audiovisual stimuli and sometimes handheld controllers to add
physical or tactile stimuli, immerse children in an absorbing virtual
environment, such as a soccer field, an ice castle, or a grocery store.
The programs can be used to engage kids in physical therapy tasks
wherever they are, or to help kids better tolerate pain or painful procedures in a hospital setting. Researchers have found, for example,
that kids engage much more willingly in strength-training exercises
when they're part of a virtual soccer game—and experience less pain
during burn treatments when a VR program gives them a magical,
snowy world to explore. As telehealth services become even more
mainstream, all of these virtual options may soon be more widely
available.[22]

Finding Comfort

Another program that is giving children increased access to effective pain management is the Comfort Ability Program, which was
created by Dr. Coakley in 2011 at Boston Children's, and is now offered at about twenty children's hospitals across the United States,
Canada, and Australia. Originally developed as a one-day, in-person
workshop run by pediatric pain psychologists, the program has now
expanded to include virtual workshops and other online resources
that teach kids with chronic pain and their parents essential pain
management techniques they can use in their daily lives. Ultimately,

the mission of the program is to connect families to the evidence-based information and skills that can help reverse the cycle of chronic pain. Since its founding, the program has grown to include disease-specific interventions (for conditions such as sickle cell disease) and a wide array of free resources, such as online health chats for adolescents and parents, and opportunities to connect virtually with pain experts. For kids without a pain clinic or pediatric pain psychologist in their area, this can be a lifeline.[23]

Like Dr. Palermo, Dr. Coakley was inspired to create this program because she recognized there was a great need to help more children faster. "When I started at the pain treatment service at Boston Children's in 2009 and looked at our clinic wait list, I saw there were about seventy patients waiting to be seen. It was mind-blowing," says Dr. Coakley. "I thought, 'My gosh, it will be years before I get through this wait list.'"

Dr. Coakley realized that, since the core teachings of pain science and cognitive behavioral therapy skills training are generally applicable to children with all types of chronic pain, it would make sense to run group workshops. In her words: "It was clear to me that how I started each course of CBT treatment was very similar whether my patient had headaches, abdominal pain, nerve pain, or disease-related pain. It didn't matter where they hurt or why they hurt because many of the fundamentals were the same. You have to teach about the neurobiological risks, pain neuroscience education, behavioral lifestyle pieces like good sleep health, and talk about how anxiety and depression fit into this." By covering these topics in a group workshop, she could provide many families simultaneously with a strong foundation from which to launch their recovery. "Importantly," she adds, "you have to do it all in a very validating and non-stigmatizing way so families feel supported and can come to understand that pain is not just a psychological problem, rather, it's a complex problem and psychology is one piece of it."

The Comfort Ability workshop is a structured program that includes one session for parents or caregivers running at the same time as another session for the kids. The goal is for a family to come away from the workshop with a shared language and shared strategies to guide a child's recovery from chronic pain. But by separating adults and kids into different spaces, the program leaders are able to target content to the specific needs of each group. "For the kids in a small group setting, they're able to learn pain management skills and build confidence that they can play an active role in managing their symptoms," says Dr. Coakley. "For the caregivers and parents, I knew we really needed time just with them because so frequently I could see that they were overwhelmed and feeling very helpless. Their children were suffering and the parents often didn't know what to do." The parent sessions, therefore, devote time to topics like how to communicate with and support a child better, and how to map out a plan for a child to return to functioning.

Fiona attended one of the earliest Comfort Ability workshops at Boston Children's, and later became a peer advisor for the program. She believes it was a pivotal moment in her treatment: "The workshop gave me tools to be active in my own recovery instead of being passive and just lying in bed and resting. It's very empowering to feel active in my own healthcare." She also "learned that it's worth sticking with the coping strategies and not giving up on them if they don't work on the first try. A lot of the strategies that worked for me in the end, like guided imagery and belly breathing, took a little practice." A bonus was that she also learned from the other kids in her group. "Everyone develops little coping strategies over the years—we've all tried the strangest things—and other kids have thought of really creative things that I've then tried and found they worked for me, too."

Beyond swapping strategies, the workshop gave Fiona a chance to connect emotionally with the other kids she met there. "I didn't know anyone else with chronic pain—adults or kids," she says. "My friends and siblings and parents all tried really hard to understand, but it's almost impossible to understand if you're not experiencing it. When I went to the workshop, I had this feeling like, 'Oh my gosh, I'm not the only one.' It was really validating to me and refreshing to feel there are other people like me, and the groups really quickly felt like a little community because we had this thing that we shared."

Dr. Coakley emphasizes that the social connections that both kids and parents gain from the workshop are invaluable. "More and more, we find that kids with chronic pain benefit from being with others who have a shared experience. These kids are scared, exhausted, struggling in school, they can't participate in the activities, and they feel alienated by their friends," says Dr. Coakley. Meeting in this safe group setting gives them permission to let their guards down, reminds them that they are not alone, and gives them hope that things can improve.

Parents, too, benefit from being in a small group setting where they can connect based on shared experience. According to Dr. Coakley, participant surveys reveal that fewer than 10 percent of parents come into the workshop expecting to gain social support from it—but almost 40 percent say afterwards that connecting with other parents of children living with pain was among the aspects of the program experience they valued most.

When the Covid-19 pandemic abruptly changed what was possible in terms of physical gatherings, Dr. Coakley worked quickly to adapt the entire workshop so it could be delivered online. While the in-person connection remains ideal, this has meant that families can still benefit from group sessions even if they can't be in the same room together. In whatever way families access resources, the most important message to remember is that help is available, and it's worth pursuing. With the increasing number of programs for children with chronic pain—both in-person and online—more kids can, and do, get better.

Chapter 11

Family Ties

*The power that parents have to affect a child's
response to pain*

Anna first began treating children with chronic pain in 2006, when she started her fellowship in pediatric psychology. She was fresh out of graduate school and optimistic about the effective tools and evidence-based treatment options that were available to kids with chronic pain—options that have only grown since. But she was disheartened to see just how drastically recurrent pain could derail the lives of children and their families. Kids who had previously been engaged in school or busy with friends and sports teams were regularly coming into Anna's office saying that they could barely make it out of bed to attend classes, that their social lives were decimated, that they could no longer take part in the activities they once loved. Anna recognized that by the time children ended up at the pain clinic their situation was often severe. While she was eager to treat her patients and help them regain a sense of normalcy in their lives, she became equally committed to figuring out how to prevent kids from spiraling into chronic pain in the first place.

Early in her clinical work, one of the most striking things Anna noticed was that the children she saw struggling with persistent pain often had parents, aunts, uncles, or grandparents with their own pain problems. Anna knew of research showing that up to 60 percent of children with chronic pain have a parent with chronic pain.[1] And she knew that scientists believed genetics were a driving force. But she saw a different way to interpret the statistics on one particularly noteworthy afternoon in the clinic. On that day, Anna remembers walking to the lobby to introduce herself to a teenager named Sarah who had been experiencing leg and hip pain for almost a year. The young girl had a brace wrapped around her knee and she sat next to her mom on the edge of a long, lime-green bench in the waiting room. Anna said hello to Sarah, and then turned to Sarah's mother who said a friendly hello but politely declined to shake hands because her shoulder had been bothering her. Then, as Anna began to lead the duo to the treatment room, Sarah stopped her, and said, "Oh, we have to wait for my grandma to get back from the restroom, but it might take her a few minutes because she has hip problems just like me." Soon enough, Anna learned that Sarah's grandmother had been using a walker since she was in her forties because of her own severe pain. After talking with the family—representing three generations—Anna couldn't shake the thought that, for Sarah's entire lifetime, her mother and her grandmother's suffering and behavior had been a central influence. Perhaps, beyond family genetics, the family environment played a critical role in the development of pain.

While this line of thought could have seemed like a path to despair—highlighting one more way in which children are set up to follow in their parents' painful footsteps—Anna saw it as an opportunity. What if she could work directly with parents who have chronic pain to prevent the future development of chronic pain in their children? Anna realized that parents tend to bring their own pain history, beliefs, behaviors, emotions, fears, and coping strategies to every interaction they have with their children around pain. Common sense would suggest that those interactions could either drive children to have healthy or unhealthy responses to pain. Perhaps a key to stopping the progression of pain in children required looking back a generation.

When Anna initially looked for research in this realm, she found surprisingly few studies on how parents' chronic pain might affect their parenting behaviors or reactions to their children's pain. There was, however, a growing body of research evaluating how parents in general respond to their children's pain, and what impact their responses could have on the kids.[2] For instance, studies have consistently shown that if parents exhibit more fear and alarm when their children are in pain (technically called catastrophizing), kids tend to view the situation as more threatening, which can add stress and subsequently ratchet up their levels of pain. In most instances, parents don't even realize they are catastrophizing, but it can be difficult to hide. It can come across through a mother's look of fear when a child falls down, in a father's worried tone of voice even while he's saying "it's going to be okay," or when a parent spends an excessive amount of time trying to soothe a child.[3] Those responses, no matter how well intentioned, can send kids the message that the pain they are experiencing is dangerous and that they can't manage it on their own. If the responses are consistent enough, the kids may then learn to engage in catastrophizing themselves, adding to their anxiety and fear and, again, making pain worse. It can be a vicious cycle.[4] But when Anna went looking for studies specifically focused on parents with chronic pain and the impact of their behaviors on the functioning of their families and the pain experiences of their children, there wasn't much out there. So Anna decided to take on those research questions and get the answers.

Learning by Observing

First, it's important to make clear that research does not show that parents are the *cause* of their children's pain problems. Rather, children experience pain in the *context* of their families. Children are keen observers of their parents' physical and emotional states, and this puts parents in a unique position to contribute to their child's understanding of pain, either directly or indirectly.

We've known since at least the 1970s, when Albert Bandura put forth his social learning theory proposing that humans learn a great deal through observation alone.[5] Although this theory was fairly radical when Bandura first articulated it, the idea is now broadly accepted that we don't always have to teach things explicitly or reward people directly for them to learn. Children in particular are highly attentive to their parents' behaviors, especially as they relate to threats, so they can learn to avoid dangerous things (such as busy streets or hot stoves) simply by watching their parents interact with the world and noticing their responses. What's more, children are likely to act on that implicit schooling by imitating the behavior that parents model, starting with such simple behaviors as eating with a fork and saying "please" and "thank you."

For decades, it was assumed that this straightforward modeling process was happening in families where a parent had chronic pain. For instance, a boy might observe his mother modeling pain (say, by rubbing her sore neck) and using a coping behavior (such as getting out the heating pad) and learn to do the same when he had a pain. But it was only recently that scientists began testing this theory and trying to measure just how much children pay attention to their parent's pain, and how they process this information.

Breeding Grounds for Chronic Pain

One of Anna's earliest studies, which she began in 2009, examined the ways in which parents with chronic pain may influence their children's perception of pain. She recruited 178 children and their parents (some of whom had chronic pain and some of whom didn't), who all completed questionnaires that asked them about their levels of pain, their responses to pain, and its frequency in their everyday lives.[6] The children in the study were all eleven to fourteen years old, the age range when chronic pain often begins. Anna discovered that the children who had a mother or father with chronic pain reported having more frequent and more intense pain themselves. Additionally, the more areas of pain that parents identified, the greater their tendency to catastrophize about their child's pain (by, for example, worrying excessively about the pain). Parents' catastrophizing was then associated with their children's catastrophizing about their own pain, which in turn influenced the kids' degree of pain-related disability. In effect, the kids had seemingly paid very close attention to their parents' pain experiences and responses and had learned from them.

A subsequent study led by Anna delved further into how parents' chronic pain might affect their parenting and their children's pain responses. The study, called the Parent and Teen Health Study, involved more than one hundred mothers and fathers (some with chronic pain and some without), each with a biological child who was eleven to fifteen years old. The parents and children completed questionnaires about pain experiences and responses, and physical and emotional health. The children also participated in specific physical activities in the lab (these included timed walks and fitness challenges, such as going back and forth from a sitting position to a standing position for one minute), and the parents with chronic pain were interviewed about their experiences parenting with chronic pain.

Here's what Anna found. Among the kids who had a parent with chronic pain (known as the high-risk group), 46 percent—almost half of the kids—said that they'd had pain weekly or more over the past three months. This was more than double the rate of pain compared to the group of kids who didn't have a parent with chronic pain (the low-risk group). Further, the parents with chronic pain tended to catastrophize about their child's pain more, and were more protective when their child had pain (for instance, they might keep their child indoors or home from school because of pain) than the parents without chronic pain. These findings confirmed the idea that parents with chronic pain may be more likely to notice and respond to their child's pain when it occurs, to interpret the pain as threatening, and to pass on this view of pain to their children.[7]

The interviews with the parents who had chronic pain were also revelatory. Many of them said they felt guilty about how their pain affected their parenting. They worried they were more impatient with their children or that their approach to discipline was less consistent because their pain often undermined their best intentions. Most of the parents also said that they had trouble being physically involved in parenting and that they missed out on some of their kids' activities. Three-quarters of these parents said that they were worried that their child would develop a problem with chronic pain.[8]

Interestingly, the children in the high-risk group were not more sensitive to pain in the lab than the kids in the low-risk group, but the high-risk kids did perform significantly worse on tests that measured physical function. This could have been due to a variety of factors. For instance, perhaps the kids were in pain during the physical tasks, or they were fearful of hurting themselves and therefore less comfortable moving, or maybe they simply weren't used to much physical activity in their household. While this study didn't capture why each of these kids didn't tend to perform well physically, it's useful to note that their pain sensitivity was not what was holding them back. And since inactivity increases the risk of chronic pain, these kids could be encouraged to move more, despite their fears or tendencies surrounding pain, which could decrease their chances of developing chronic pain.[9]

Anna's research has also been informed by data from a large, ongoing population study out of Norway that has collected health information from over 125,000 people (including adults and adolescents) since the 1980s.[10] Using this data set, researchers have been able to look at how chronic pain conditions are linked within families and determine the proportion of the connections that are due to genetic similarities. In the case of chronic pain conditions, researchers found that the links between parents and children cannot be explained completely by genetics.[11] Rather, a child's family environment also significantly influences whether that child will develop pain problems. This finding was underscored when researchers were able to compare how children fared depending on which parent lived with them, which helped to separate behavioral influences from genetics. This research strengthened Anna's desire to keep studying parents with pain and to find ways to reduce the risk of pain problems in their children. While there's not yet a great deal that science can do to alter the genetic risk for chronic pain, there are ways that clinicians can support parents in pain so that they are less likely to perpetuate a cycle of chronic pain in their kids. (See the end of this chapter for tips.)

Parenting in Pain

As Anna was studying parents in pain, Rachel was living it in her everyday life as a mother with chronic back pain raising two young children, Lena and Annika. The pain was not new to Rachel but the strain and stress that it added to motherhood was a new kind of suffering. Rachel had been diagnosed with scoliosis (a curvature of the spine) at eight years old and had worn a brace under her clothes from then until age sixteen in an effort to correct the course of her S-shaped spine as she grew. While the treatment did initially steady her spine's trajectory, ultimately the rigid plastic brace couldn't contain the worsening curve. As Rachel's scoliosis progressed during adulthood, pain permeated the taut muscles surrounding her unruly spine. Spasms, pangs, and aches riddled her back, shoulders, and neck, and triggered frequent headaches. Still, the pain was manageable, and before having children, Rachel didn't fully comprehend how her pain would affect her parenting.

Yet one of the many things Rachel learned when she became a mother, to Lena in 2008, was that parenting is demanding physical work. This is particularly true for the millions of parents with chronic pain.[12] Standing and rocking a baby to sleep, hoisting a toddler into and out of a highchair, and lugging a stroller up the stairs day in and day out can be arduous tasks. For Rachel, her body buckled under the strain. Back spasms often kept her from standing or walking for long stretches, neck stiffness stopped her from turning her head, and shoulder pangs sometimes made it impossible to lift an arm. Although she tried many different approaches to quell the pain with varying success—including physical therapy, acupuncture, massage, and over-the-counter anti-inflammatory medications—the pain remained. And when Annika was born in 2011, the physical load increased.

What frustrated Rachel the most, however, was not the pain she experienced; it was how the pain seemed to rob her of being the best mother she could be for her kids. There were countless days when she couldn't lift her preschooler onto the jungle gym or carry her toddler on her hip, yet there were her children, reaching up their arms, unable to comprehend why their mother refused them. There were also too many instances when Rachel felt her stamina and patience dwindling as her pain flared.

Like so many of the mothers Anna includes in her studies, Rachel felt guilty and worried that she was causing her children to suffer. Further, as a health journalist, she'd read the growing body of research that Anna and her peers were producing, and the science seemed to confirm Rachel's deepest fears. Evidence showed that in families where a parent has chronic pain, their children are at increased risk for developing chronic pain—and also at greater risk for behavioral issues, anxiety, and depression than children whose parents are pain-free.[13]

One study led by Wendy Umberger, a nursing professor at Kent State University in Ohio, painted a particularly grim picture of what might become of Rachel's relationship with her children, and it haunted her. The researchers in the study interviewed a group of thirty adolescents who grew up with parents experiencing chronic pain. In many cases, the children felt their parents were uninvolved physically and emotionally—even irritable, hostile, and unpredictable. Because of this, the children often hid their needs and true feelings from their parents, living in fear of upsetting their parents or worsening their pain. Many took on caretaking roles before they were ready to do so. Some questioned whether they were to blame for their parents' suffering. These family dynamics spawned a variety of heartbreaking outcomes for the children, some of whom became perfectionists, learned to retreat in silence, or turned to substance abuse.[14]

Worried that this could be her own children's fate, Rachel made learning more about it a part of her work as a journalist. Her reporting and writing pulled her deeper into the literature relating to parental chronic pain and how it may affect children.[15] But, to her relief, she learned it doesn't have to determine a family's future.

What's more, the latest research (some of it led by Anna) continues to provide reasons to be hopeful. For example, Anna's ongoing work includes following a cohort of four hundred mothers with chronic pain and their children for a total of three years, as the kids enter adolescence.[16] By studying how these mothers' behaviors affect their children's physical and mental health, Anna is assessing potential ways to intervene that could prevent children from "inheriting" pain problems, anxiety, or depression. She is also analyzing whether and how children of various ages and genders respond differently to their parents' pain, a line of work that could pave the way for future research on how to tailor interventions for specific groups of children.

Anna is also among an increasing number of scientists around the world who are studying the impact of parental chronic pain on children. Up-and-coming pediatric pain researchers like Amanda Stone at Vanderbilt University Medical Center in Nashville (who was a graduate student under Dr. Lynn Walker's mentorship and a postdoctoral fellow in Anna's lab), Kristen Higgins at Dalhousie University in Halifax, and Elke Van Lierde, a graduate student at Ghent University in Ghent, Belgium, are carrying out important work that will add to our understanding of chronic pain across generations.[17] Anna and her colleagues are determined to break the intergenerational cycle of chronic pain and find answers for the many families who could benefit.

Key Tips for Parents with Chronic Pain

Though science may indicate that the odds are against parents with pain problems, researchers have identified a variety of positive actions parents can take to prevent the progression of chronic pain in their children and increase resilience.

- **Take care of yourself.** Managing your chronic pain while taking care of your children can feel exhausting and overwhelming. Know that addressing your own physical and emotional well-being will also benefit your child. But keep in mind that caring for yourself does not mean chronic pain should become your central identity. While pain demands attention and getting good treatment can feel like a full-time job, remember that you are not defined by your pain. You are a parent. Perhaps, too, you are a spouse, a son or daughter, a friend. You may have a career or hobbies. Remember to engage with the people and activities that bring meaning and joy to your life, and make you so much more than your pain.
- **Try not to catastrophize about your own pain or your child's.** This is easier said than done, but once you realize that assuming the worst is a tendency that actually intensifies pain, it becomes more possible to rein it in. For starters, pause to identify catastrophizing thoughts when they

pop up (like "I will never get better" or "There is no way this treatment will work"), because this can be a signal to reframe your thought process. Make an effort to learn more about pain and how it works in the body; pain education often helps people view their discomfort as less threatening, which can reduce the worry and anxiety that can lead to catastrophizing thoughts. (In fact, we hope that this book is already helping to demystify what pain is and isn't.)

There are also education programs for adults that can reduce pain catastrophizing. Beth Darnall, a pain psychologist at Stanford University, has developed an innovative two-hour course that teaches adults how to identify catastrophizing thoughts in the moment and immediately act to tamp them down.[18] The course, which is increasingly available across the country, elucidates how cognitive behavioral strategies, such as reframing your perspective, deep breathing, and muscle relaxation, can reduce anxiety and rumination about pain. Chances are, if you learn to worry less about your own pain, you will also worry less about your child's.

- **Label your pain and coping strategies out loud.** While clinicians would not recommend that parents moan daily about their pain, it is helpful to let your kids know what you're experiencing, when necessary, so that they can understand your behavior. This is important because many of the best coping strategies that adults tend to employ may not be obvious to children. For example, instead of hiding the fact that you're struggling with a headache, let your child know you're not feeling well by saying, "I think I feel a headache coming on." Then model a positive coping strategy by saying, "I'm going to take a bath and relax so I can keep this headache from getting worse." If your kids know what you're experiencing, they won't be left wondering why you seemed upset or left the room to be alone. Similarly, if you often deal with back pain by, say, taking a short walk, clue your children into your approach. They'll learn that pain doesn't have to elicit alarm bells, and can be managed calmly.

· **Model a multidisciplinary approach.** As Chapter 10 explains, for many people with chronic pain, there is no magic pill or one modality that cures all. Rather, most people benefit from a range of treatments that may include cognitive behavioral therapy, physical therapy, good nutrition, stress relief, and medication as needed. For parents in pain, consider what pain management behaviors you show your children. Ideally, you are showing them coping strategies beyond taking medication. You might show your children that you make an effort to walk daily or get enough sleep so that you can minimize your pain. Rachel, for instance, eventually sought out a scoliosis-specific physical therapy called Schroth, which has significantly helped her reduce her pain. Her kids (who are now old enough to understand more) know that when Rachel's doing her Schroth exercises, she's putting in the time to strengthen her body and minimize pain. She hopes her children will internalize this approach and follow it if necessary.

· **Don't focus too much on your pain.** Research has shown that when parents fixate on their own pain, it can make pain worse for their kids. In two separate laboratory studies, parents were told to put their hand in very cold water (a classic pain test), and either exaggerate or minimize their expression of pain while their children watched. Next, the kids underwent the same cold water test and then rated their pain levels. It turned out that the level of pain that the parents showed influenced how much pain and anxiety their child experienced themselves, with girls in particular being vulnerable to experiencing more pain when it was exaggerated by a parent.[19] The takeaway: If you make a big deal about pain, your kids are likely to follow suit.

· **Keep yourself—and your family—moving.** If you're able, model movement and exercise, and play physically with your kids. If you're not able, don't worry. You don't need to be your kids' baseball coach to bring physical activity into their lives. Even from the sidelines, there are plenty of ways to help your kids keep moving, which may lower their risk of developing chronic pain. For instance, encourage them to sign up for school sports or dance classes, assign them physical chores around the house (like taking out the trash), let them play outside with friends or neighbors, and consider asking other adult family members or friends to take your kids to the park, go for a hike, or shoot hoops in the driveway. If you find yourself feeling anxious about letting your children play sports, or you fear that their physical activity may cause pain, don't let your worries stop your kids. Ultimately, if they're physically (and socially) active, and have permission to be kids, they'll be more likely to grow into fulfilled and happy adults.

- **Don't forget to have fun.** When pain feels intolerable and managing the day-to-day feels oppressive, it can be easy to forget about the simple and enjoyable things we can do with our kids. Playing board games, baking or cooking, reading books aloud, watching movies, and doing crafts are all opportunities to share positive moments with your children. Making time for these types of activities will let your kids know that even if you have pain, you can still enjoy your life, and your family as a whole can weather stressful times and still have fun together. If you're having trouble connecting with your kids, or want help managing pain and parenting, seek out a pain psychologist or a pediatric psychologist if you can.

- **Give yourself a break.** There is no question that tackling these tasks may feel overwhelming. Parenting under typical circumstances is hard, and parenting while managing your pain or your child's pain can feel impossible. So be kind to yourself, and try not to feel guilty for doing the best that you can. Make time for your own sleep, exercise, meals, and relaxation—and know that the better you feel, the better off both you and your family will be. It's taken Rachel and Anna a long time to learn that, and while we don't always remember to take our own advice, we hope that you do.

Chapter 12

The Invisible Burden of Pain

When stigma and bias lead to isolation and
depression, social support can help

When Jillian was fourteen years old she was in a minor car accident and suffered whiplash, which developed into severe pain and stiffness in her neck. Immediately after the accident, her pediatrician gave her a neck brace to wear. At first, Jillian, a petite girl, was embarrassed and self-conscious about wearing the clunky brace at school. But she was also relieved, in a sense, that the brace served as a signal to her friends and teachers that she was injured, so she didn't have to explain herself when she couldn't participate in activities.

After those first few weeks, though, Jillian's doctor concluded the brace wasn't helping, and instructed her to stop wearing it. Now, without the visible sign of her pain, few people around Jillian understood why she walked slowly, acted tired, and didn't hang out much after school. After three months of aggravating neck pain that was interfering with her ability to sleep and concentrate, Jillian was referred to Anna. Not only was the pain overtaking her life, but she felt disconnected from her friends, isolated, and judged in a way she'd never experienced before. In one of her first sessions with Anna she said, "Sometimes I wish I still had the brace, because then at least people would know that something was wrong with me."

For Jillian, and most children with chronic pain, one of the hardest aspects of managing their condition is the fact that other people don't understand it, or simply don't believe it's real. Pain is invisible, it is silent, and, of course, it is subjective, which can make children in chronic pain feel like they are living in a dystopian world all their own. Without a single diagnostic test to assess for the presence of pain, even medical professionals may dismiss kids' suffering and invalidate their experiences. In many cases, children's own parents have a hard time believing.

Researchers estimate that at least 40 percent of children with chronic pain have experienced dismissal or disbelief from adults, most frequently from medical providers and parents.[1] This leaves kids with pain particularly vulnerable to stigma—the experience of being singled out and judged for having an attribute that is considered undesirable by society. And this can have devastating, even life-threatening, consequences in the context of healthcare. Researchers have found that people with chronic pain conditions are often devalued, discredited, stereotyped, rejected, and even ostracized. This, in turn, can lead to delayed diagnosis, treatment bias, and poor health outcomes. Notably, pain-related stigma is more likely to happen to girls and women and to racial and ethnic minorities than to white boys and men, as we'll discuss later in this chapter.[2]

While pain-related stigma has been well documented in adults, there are fewer studies on stigma and chronic pain in children. But recent research in the area is confirming what many kids with chronic pain have long experienced: they often feel stigmatized by medical providers, parents, other family members, friends, and school staff.[3] This can then fuel many of the other negative outcomes that afflict children with chronic pain, including inadequate care, depression, social isolation, and academic struggles. In essence, the weight of stigma can burden children in nearly every realm of their life, making every challenge harder to bear.[4]

Emily's Story: Facing Skepticism

Emily and her mother, Susan, have spent twenty years confronting other people's skepticism about the Crohn's disease afflicting Emily and the agonizing pain this severe inflammatory bowel disease causes. From the earliest days of Emily's illness, when she began to develop mysterious fevers and infections during her kindergarten year, the family felt second-guessed by teachers and other parents— even their pediatrician at the time. "Emily never looked the part," remembers Susan, who is also a nurse. "She would often get up in the morning and look and feel fine, and then as the day wore on she would become feverish, tired, and uncomfortable, but other people wouldn't see that. To the rest of the world, she seemed perky." Emily's bright disposition disguised the pain she was feeling.

It took a year for the family to get a referral to appropriate specialists in New York City, near their home in the suburbs, and even then the doctors underestimated the gravity of Emily's illness. "She would walk into the doctor's office smiling, and she never seemed sick," explains Susan. "In the course of testing her, the medical team even called in a psychiatric consult to interview me for Munchausen syndrome by proxy, thinking that maybe I was making this all up!" It was only after Emily's blood work came back and she underwent a colonoscopy that the specialists recognized Emily was suffering from a serious condition.

The battle to be understood, however, has been a long-lasting one, and it has influenced Emily's treatment. For example, when she was eight years old, she went to a five-day sleepaway camp for children with Crohn's. Susan was at first hesitant to let Emily go, but then agreed to allow it because Emily's doctor was running the camp and would be onsite. Three days into the camp, after seeing Emily's ups and downs with gastrointestinal pain and fevers, day and night, the doctor called Susan to say, "I think we're really undertreating Emily; we'll have to make some adjustments when we get back."

Finally, Susan thought, *someone understands.* "No one was believing how severe it was," she says. "It's like, there was this piece of paper with lab work, and then there was this child and how she would present to the world—and it didn't add up for doctors."

Susan and Emily, now in her mid-twenties, have since become adept at advocating for the treatment Emily needs, but getting to this point wasn't easy. "She's suffered from a lot of pain, from intense and constant abdominal cramping, and when I think back, the pain was completely ignored. No one addressed it," says Susan. "It was always 'let's look at the hemoglobin and her sedimentation rate or her C-reactive protein'—it was about the medical and physical." When Susan compares her daughter's childhood experience with her husband's recent inpatient hospital stay for surgery, she marvels at the differences. "Every time someone came into the room to see my husband during his stay, the first thing they said was, 'Tell me your pain from 0 to 10,'" says Susan. "That was never asked of Emily, ever. Never ever."

Gender Bias in Pain Management

Research sheds light on Susan and Emily's experience, which is not uncommon today. Not only is pain often overlooked in kids, pain is more often dismissed in girls and women than in boys and men.[5]

A recent large review of scientific literature shows this gender bias in healthcare, especially as it pertains to chronic pain.[6] Of course, there *are* biological differences in males and females that influence their perceptions of pain—but there are also societal factors that influence how people of all genders perceive and report pain, and how healthcare providers respond to them.[7] The result is that girls in pain are more likely to be viewed as emotional, hysterical, and faking the pain, while boys are more likely to be viewed as stoic and brave. As for children who identify as nonbinary or transgender, researchers are just beginning to understand how biases may affect their pain management.[8] In general, however, it's already clear that getting appropriate healthcare as a nonbinary or transgender individual can be an uphill battle.

Persistent stereotyped gender norms do a disservice to children of all genders seeking appropriate pain management. Fortunately, however, new research on gender bias and stigma in healthcare is offering hope for improvements to the status quo. There is also a call from scientists for more female representation in both human and animal studies on pain so that sex and gender will be better integrated into our collective understanding of pain.[9]

In Emily's case, she did eventually find clinicians she trusts and who listen to her. As with many young patients, she learned, as she got older, to value her own instincts, to advocate for herself within the healthcare system, and to seek out practitioners who would respond to her needs. Now, as a young adult, she is a medical social worker. Her mom says she was determined to work in a hospital so she could "give back" some of the knowledge she's acquired over the years. No doubt, she is one of a new generation of hospital staffers who can help patients feel seen and be heard.

Racial Bias in Pain Management

The role of racial bias and stigma in healthcare is undeniable. A large body of research has documented centuries of racial inequities in medical care for Black Americans and other minorities, dating back to the days of slavery.[10] There has been a concerted effort to address these disparities—particularly in the last thirty-five years since the US Department of Health and Human Services issued its landmark "Report of the Secretary's Task Force on Black and Minority Health."[11] But parity by any measure has not been achieved. Due in part to legislative, socioeconomic, and cultural factors, adults and children of color in the United States tend to have less access to high-quality healthcare and are more likely to suffer from—and succumb to—chronic illnesses at younger ages than white people.[12] This tragic inequality has taken center stage most recently with the Covid-19 pandemic, with its disproportionate impacts on Americans of color.

The disparities and stigma also exist in the realm of pain management.[13] Research shows that pain is frequently underestimated and undertreated in Black, Native American, and Hispanic people (and other minorities) compared to white people. Studies reveal that adults and children of color are less likely than their white counterparts to be given pain medications in emergency departments and after surgery—and when pain medications are prescribed, they are given in lower quantities.[14]

A 2015 study of nearly a million children with appendicitis, led by Monika Goyal, a pediatric emergency medicine specialist at Children's National Hospital in Washington, DC, revealed that children of different races received unequal pain treatment. Black children with appendicitis who reported moderate pain in the emergency department were less likely to receive analgesics than white children with appendicitis, and Black children who reported severe pain were less likely to receive opioids.[15]

"There are a lot of data that support treating the pain in children with appendicitis—and treating it with opioids—because appendicitis can be quite painful, and there's really no downside to the use of opioids in the acute care setting," explains Dr. Goyal, who is also an associate professor of pediatrics and emergency medicine at George Washington University. "But we found that even after we accounted for severity of pain, Black children had a lower likelihood of receiving any type of analgesia—and also specifically opioid analgesia—than white children."

The reasons for this are varied and require further study, says Dr. Goyal, but she believes the disparities in pain management have largely to do with implicit racial bias and how that relates to the opioid epidemic. "We are no doubt suffering through an opioid epidemic right now and a lot of that is due to overuse of opioids, but again, there are very strong data showing that opioids do not lead to addiction when used to treat acute, self-limited painful conditions such as appendicitis," says Dr. Goyal. Further, the tendency to withhold opioids from children of color—as compared to white children—is especially misguided based on what we know about the opioid epidemic. "When you think about who is being more affected by the opioid epidemic, the data show that the opioid epidemic is much worse in white populations. Yet we as clinicians make mistaken assumptions about drug-seeking behavior or opioid misuse in Black and brown populations that leads to the undertreatment of pain in minority children."

A subsequent study led by Dr. Goyal, published in 2020, focused on children who went to the emergency department for fractures.[16]

Again, the study found that Black children and other minorities were less likely to receive opioids and less likely to achieve optimal pain relief than their white counterparts. "Many people thought that these disparities didn't happen in pediatrics and that it was specific to an adult population," says Dr. Goyal. "But now that we've shown that these racial and ethnic disparities do indeed exist even in the care of children, it speaks volumes to the bias and structural racism within the healthcare system."

Other research shows that shocking misconceptions persist among medical practitioners about biological differences between Black and white people. In a 2016 study published in the journal *Proceedings of the National Academy of Sciences,* researchers surveyed 222 white medical students and residents, and found that about half of them held false beliefs related to how Black people perceive pain versus white people. For instance, almost 60 percent of the white medical students and residents sampled held the erroneous belief that Black people have thicker skin than white people do. About 11 percent believed that Black people's nerve endings are less sensitive than white people's. The study authors concluded that, even in this day and age, beliefs that date back to slavery about racial biological differences continue to exercise their hold over some healthcare professionals. Those beliefs contribute to the perception that Black people feel less pain than do white people, which can lead to inadequate treatment for Black people experiencing pain.[17] "It's amazing how, even unconsciously, some of that implicit bias has seeped into people's beliefs," says Dr. Goyal.

A growing number of scientists are studying the role of bias in healthcare, and proposing ways to mitigate it, including by offering more education on race, stereotypes, and bias in medical schools.

Janice A. Sabin, a research associate professor of biomedical informatics and medical education at the University of Washington School of Medicine in Seattle, is one such scientist. Her research and courses aim to reduce healthcare disparities among minority populations.[18] "As a nation, we must continue to reckon with the lingering history of racism in medicine," Dr. Sabin recently wrote. "Dramatically reducing, and perhaps even eliminating racial and ethnic disparities in pain treatment is an attainable goal—and a moral imperative."[19]

One way to achieve more parity is to highlight the problem. "So much of this is implicit, and many practitioners' first reaction is to think that this doesn't happen in their care setting. So providing the data can be very eye-opening," says Dr. Goyal. She recommends that physicians take a test called the Implicit Association Test, which measures the attitudes, beliefs, and stereotypes people hold.[20] "If the test reveals you have anti-Black implicit bias, for instance, it doesn't necessarily mean you're a racist, but what's really important is being aware of that bias, and being able to use that awareness and take it with you every time you're treating a patient," she says.

Dr. Goyal also notes that more racial and ethnic diversity among physicians could help reduce racial and ethnic inequalities in healthcare, including when there are potential language barriers. "The medical community, specifically the physician community, is not very diverse, and we need to be doing a better job in medicine so that the people who are representing the medical community are representative of the population they're serving," she says. Dr. Goyal thinks there has been progress on that front in the last few years as movements such as White Coats for Black Lives (a nonprofit run by medical students aimed at dismantling racism in medicine) have moved more to the forefront.[21] But there is still a long way to go. "I'm hopeful," says Dr. Goyal, "that in the next five years the composition of physicians will be much more diverse than it has been historically."

Adrian's Story: Sickle Cell Anemia and Invisible Scars

Adrian Williams, a patient-care advocate in Washington, DC, has felt this inequity on a visceral level. He was born in the 1960s with sickle cell anemia, also called sickle cell disease, which is an inherited red blood cell disorder that can cause organ and tissue damage as well as excruciating pain. The illness most commonly affects Black people, and research shows that stigma plays a significant role in the lives of those with sickle cell disease, including children.[22]

Adrian was raised by his aunt and uncle, who were extremely loving but who didn't have access to health insurance until the passage of Medicaid in 1965. "We were very lower-middle class," says Adrian, who has a warm and distinguished demeanor. "I was a minority child with limited access to great care, and my aunt and uncle weren't college-educated or super-savvy with respect to getting to those medical resources in a timely manner." As a result, he didn't get diagnosed with sickle cell disease until he was about five years old, and he didn't receive regular treatment for several years of his childhood, which meant that he often suffered unbearable episodes of pain with little recourse.

His earliest memories of that pain center around his experiences with intermittent sickle cell crises, which happen when oxygen-carrying red blood cells (normally soft and round) become sickle-shaped and clump together, making it difficult for those red blood cells to flow through the small blood vessels of the body. This blockage of blood and oxygen can cause debilitating pain in the chest, abdomen, joints, bones—essentially, everywhere. When those episodes would occur, Adrian would spend days in his bed in what he describes as a "dark pit—this three- to five-day prison sentence of pain. There's no rescue, there's no reprieve."

The over-the-counter medications available to Adrian in the 1960s stood no chance against the torrent of pain, so he remembers his aunt and uncle desperately trying to help him through any means available to them. They rocked his bed, propped him onto pillows, tried ice, then heat, lots of blankets, then no blankets—and when all else failed, they gave him a damp rag to bite down on. "They were definitely there with me, and very attentive," says Adrian, "but just watching something you can't really stop."

Without any substantial physical relief, Adrian trained his mind to escape. He would imagine himself leaving his body, flying above his room, above his neighborhood, and hovering overhead so he could look down on his world from an aerial view. "That's been the hallmark of my survival, the ability of my mind to transport my body in pain and go somewhere else," he says. His own instinctual self-taught guided imagery lessened the torture, but not enough.

"You can imagine the psychological damage that can do. You're forever changed when you experience one episode of that, much less reoccurring episodes of that," says Adrian. The unpredictability of the episodes compounded the trauma. Adrian describes in vivid detail the moments when a pain crisis would strike:

> I'd literally be in the middle of doing something—I could be sleeping, or on vacation, or about to go to prom—and I'd feel this heightening of my blood pressure, and then my breath would get shallow, and I'd start to pant. And once you hear the alarm in your head, you know what's coming. The pain would go from two to four to six within about an hour. It's like a thief in the night. It just taps you on the shoulder, "Hey, I'm here." The odds of you grabbing it,

or pushing it the other way are remote. So you think, "Do I need to get home?" "Do I need to go to the hospital right away?" Panic.

Around age eleven, Adrian learned about an infusion center at Georgetown University Hospital in DC, where he began to go when he felt a pain crisis coming on. The medical team there would administer oxygen and IV fluids and analgesics (including opioids, when needed), and if he could make it to the clinic within about an hour of the pain's onset, they could halt the episode within a few hours rather than a few days. It was a turning point for him.

As Adrian grew into young adulthood and became more adept at understanding his treatment needs, he also became aware that hospital staff began to view him, and treat him differently. Being a Black man did not serve him as well as being a curly-haired little boy had. "I didn't encounter overt racism in healthcare until I was a teenager, when I went to a hospital where they didn't know me," says Adrian. In that instance, he walked into the emergency department, and despite being well dressed and obviously knowledgeable about his disease, he was accused of being a drug addict in search of narcotics. He wasn't given the pain treatment he needed in time, and that visit ended up being the longest hospitalization he's experienced.

Andrew Campbell, director of the sickle cell program at Children's National Hospital in DC, has led discussion groups with Black men with sickle cell disease. He says that almost all of them have had experiences of providers simply not listening to them or not believing that their requests for opioid pain medication were justified. "They've described the experience of screaming in pain in the emergency room and even getting security called on them or thrown out of the ER because the providers have a poor understanding of the pain and cannot believe the patients could be in that much pain," he says. "Part of it is a lack of understanding about sickle cell disease, and part of it is bias and racism."

As Dr. Goyal found in her work, the opioid crisis in the United States has made it harder for some patients to receive the treatments they need. "Patients with sickle cell disease are being lumped into a [drug-abusing] category unfairly because there's an opioid crisis," says Dr. Campbell. This in turn, causes providers to limit opioid prescriptions to both adults and children with sickle cell disease. "There are providers who mistakenly believe that if you give opioids to children with sickle cell disease they're going to have problems with the medications as an adult, and there's just very little evidence of that. But what's happening is, we're getting a lot of undertreated pain for patients with sickle cell disease."

Adrian believes he is lucky because it wasn't the norm for him to be turned away at the emergency department, but he is highly aware of the biases and stigmatization that many minority patients with sickle cell disease regularly endure in the healthcare system.[23] "Patients with sickle cell will often try to look good and present themselves in a way that gives them a greater chance of getting expert care," says Adrian. He adds that for him, having to deal with that extra burden on top of the disease has added to his anxiety and pain—and has at times eroded his trust in medical providers and in people in general.

"You have to rely on yourself," says Adrian. And he has. In his thirties, he took it upon himself to completely transform his diet, lifestyle, and mindset. He shifted to a vegan diet, made time for regular exercise, and began actively practicing mindfulness, acceptance, and relaxation techniques. He credits this multidisciplinary approach with drastically reducing his pain. The last sickle cell crisis he had that required hospitalization was ten years ago. He now speaks publicly about wellness and runs an online community called "Wellness Revolution Now," which he hopes will help other people avoid some of the trauma he's experienced. He still can't quite believe that he's achieved a sense of normalcy in his life—and a freedom from severe pain—that he used to only dream about. But the invisible scars he carries have been harder to shake. "Now that I'm on the other side of that equation, it hasn't left me for one minute what psychological torment that place is," says Adrian. "I'm still a restless sleeper to this day from the fear of that pain. Even though I've been healthy all these years, the fear of that keeps me up at night. It's like that tap on your shoulder, 'Here I am.' That keeps me up at night still. Still."

School Challenges

Outside of the healthcare setting, one of the biggest challenges for children with chronic pain is being able to attend school consistently and keep up academically. Research shows that children with chronic pain are about five times more likely to miss more than fifteen days of school in a year than children without pain.[24] On average, kids with chronic pain are absent about one-third of school days.[25] Missing school and falling behind in assignments because of pain and medical visits only compounds children's already high stress levels. In Chapter 7 we met Mina, whose inability to study because of headaches caused her to go from being a straight-A student to nearly failing out of school. The disappointment and anxiety this causes for children typically drives the cycle of pain and stress.

Kids like Mina often have a very hard time explaining their need for help, and even when they do ask for accommodations, in many cases, teachers and administrators don't seem to understand. Some even pass judgment. In one survey of school nurses, almost half of them said that children had come to them complaining of pain who in their opinion were faking it or trying to get attention.[26] While research has shown that teachers are more likely to be responsive and accommodating to students in pain when they provide medical evidence or medical records about their illness, for many children with chronic pain conditions, clear medical evidence simply isn't available, and in these cases teachers may be less sympathetic and less likely to grant accommodations.[27]

Susan found that it was necessary for her to meet with Emily's teachers each year to explain to them what Crohn's disease was and how it affected Emily, so that they could be sensitive to her limitations and be aware that she may need to be absent. In high school, Emily was able to arrange her classes so that she could sometimes arrive at school later, which was often a necessity on days when her pain and gastrointestinal upset prevented her from leaving the house in the morning. Emily also tended to gravitate to at least one teacher, counselor, or school nurse who "got it," so that she felt she had some support at school. Finding an understanding adult at school can be instrumental for many kids. That ally can make it much more likely that a child with a pain condition will get back to school.

For Emily, getting to school, even for a half day, significantly improved her sense of normalcy and belonging. "Seeing her resilience even kept me going," remembers Susan. "On days when she was ill but wanted to go to school anyway, I used my child as my role model. I'd want to stay in the school parking lot and wait for her, but when I'd see my child braving through I'd realize: I have to move forward, too."

As determined as Emily was, though, it was sometimes untenable for her to get to school regularly. For instance, there were months at a time when Emily needed what is called a peripherally inserted central catheter—a PICC line—to provide her with round-the-clock intravenous nutrition and medication. This required her to stay home from school, and in those instances she was able to transition to home-schooling with the help of tutors. Other kids who can't make it to school also move to online school—but while these options can give children much-needed flexibility they also further separate them from their peers. This then reduces kids' chances of keeping up with friendships or forming new ones during a time when social support is critical in their development. (The importance of maintaining regular school connections—for children's social and emotional health and for academic engagement—has been made acutely clear to millions of families during the Covid-19 pandemic, which caused the entire country, and much of the world, to resort to online distance learning.)

Social Struggles: Isolated Whether You're There or Not

Although many people may think of the social aspects of kids' lives as a minor component of their overall health, feeling connected is critical to physical and mental well-being. What's more, when children begin to feel disconnected, this can also cause them to fear going to school and other social settings like parties and after-school activities. "It was really hard with friends," says Susan, who found it heartbreaking to watch friends come in and out of Emily's life over the years. "The unpredictability of being able to keep playdates or go to parties made it even harder. After a while it seemed that, even on the days that Emily was feeling well enough to go to a birthday party, she wouldn't want to go," says Susan, who believes that Emily developed social anxiety after years of being unable to maintain social ties.

Emily's struggles are common for kids with chronic pain and illness. Research shows that these children are more likely to be bullied and to have fewer friends.[28] Mina (who dealt with headaches, as described in Chapter 7), says that she didn't have many friends at school, partly "because I was never there. And when I was there, I didn't want to talk to anybody because I hurt really bad, or I was tired, or all of the above." Studies also demonstrate that, even apart from the pain that kids feel, social challenges engender anxiety and depression and prevent children from going to school and performing well academically.[29]

Anna remembers working with one teenage girl who had been absent for many days during the middle of the school year due to severe back pain. When she finally got back to school, after physical therapy had helped alleviate her pain, she was devastated by the new social landscape. She burst into tears in Anna's office and explained that when she first started missing school, some friends had texted her and kept in touch, but the texts began to fizzle the longer she was gone. Now that she was back, no one seemed to acknowledge her, even by saying "hi" in the hallways. "It's like I died. Everyone has just moved on with their lives," she said. The peer problems led to mild depression, which made it even more difficult for her to get back to school and her routine.

Even when friends do keep in touch, kids with chronic pain may feel they no longer have enough common ground with each other. "It's hard because I wasn't able to go out all the time and do the crazy things my friends wanted to do," says Mina. "The friends I've known since before my headaches, they'd talk about their problems and I just couldn't relate. The friend would say, 'Oh, I was asked out by three people last week—that's so rough.' And I'm thinking, 'Oh, I barely got out of bed today.'" Mina is thankful that she had one or two good friends with whom she could identify and who did try to understand where she was coming from, but she says, "it's kind of hard to imagine having a constant headache for two years."

Adrian remembers wanting to fit in as a child and trying to pretend he felt fine, but that effort took a toll. "When you're young, you're just trying to be like everyone else, to be normal, and that's a lot of weight," he says. "Pretending is a weight. You get to that place where it's you, you, and you. No one understands and you can't explain it well enough. You find that even in a room full of people you are alone—even amongst your family you are alone, because no one has experienced this stuff like you have experienced, or has the fears that accompany it like you have."

There are no easy ways to alleviate these profound feelings of isolation that so many children with chronic pain experience, but there is evidence that even a single meaningful friendship or connection can make a big difference.[30] Both Mina and Emily found friends at summer camps, which gave them some of the peer support they often lacked at school. Many other kids end up finding like-minded friends at support groups for kids who have similar conditions. Numerous patient advocacy foundations also run summer camps for children with particular healthcare needs.

Emily even figured out a place for herself at school by becoming the scorekeeper for the boys' basketball team in high school. "She desperately wanted to be a part of something," says Susan. "She wasn't able to be on a sports team but, as the scorekeeper, she made friends with all these boys, and she felt like she belonged." One of the highlights of "normalcy," as Susan calls it, was when Emily went to the prom. "I remember taking her to the store and watching her try on dresses and feeling like it was such a gift that she was getting to go to the prom. She just didn't have that regular stuff. And that was regular stuff."

Unfortunately, as much as parents may try, they can't make friends for their children. But they can help guide them. They can also work with a school counselor or psychologist to help kids gain the skills and confidence that they need to face these problems and get reconnected with peers.

The Intersection of Pain, Isolation, Depression, and Anxiety

Though estimates vary widely, research shows that up to 79 percent of children with chronic pain experience anxiety, and up to 43 percent experience depression, which can include thoughts of self-harm or suicide.[31] Much of the variability in these estimates is likely due to the fact that it can be difficult to assess symptoms of anxiety and depression in children, especially those with chronic pain.[32] The reason for this is that, when kids are dealing with a chronic pain condition in addition to feelings of isolation, it can be hard for parents, and even clinicians, to disentangle which symptoms are related to pain versus anxiety or depression.[33] Anna often talks with parents of teens who've noticed that their child is increasingly irritated with family members and spending more time alone or in bed, but who aren't sure if this is their child's way of coping with pain, or if it signals depression, or if it's typical teenager behavior—or it's a combination of all three.

In these instances, it's a good idea to talk with your child about how they're feeling. If your child won't open up, talk with your child's healthcare provider, pain team, or counselor (whichever resources you have available). Even if your child is dealing with minor anxiety or depression, it should be addressed; even lower levels of depressed mood and negative thinking can make it more difficult for children to cope with pain.

In fact, depression and chronic pain problems may be more closely related than scientists once thought. Thanks to large data sets compiled on adolescents, we know that prevalences of both depression and chronic pain rise rapidly beginning in early adolescence. The studies also show that some mental health problems, including depression and anxiety, are likely to predate the onset of chronic pain problems, such as headaches, chronic back pain, and neck pain.[34] This suggests that during the teen years in particular, having depression and anxiety may actually increase kids' risk for developing chronic pain in the first place.

Other recent studies highlight that the genetic patterns associated with depression are also associated with chronic pain conditions, and that the genetic overlap tends to cluster in families.[35] In other words, the underlying genetics that may predispose a child to developing depressive symptoms may also predispose the child to developing chronic pain. While these findings may seem overwhelmingly negative, they may help identify kids who can be targeted early with interventions to prevent depression and pain symptoms before they start.

Tackling Stigma and Improving Well-Being

Confronting the stigma, ignorance, and bias associated with chronic pain can sometimes feel like a never-ending battle. So it's helpful for families to remember that they don't always need to take on the fight. Instead, it can be eye-opening for kids to find something outside of their pain that can strengthen them and increase their independence and competence—all core developmental tasks of childhood and adolescence that often get thwarted by chronic pain.[36]

How to Navigate School Absences

For many children with pain, going to school every day and keeping up with their studies may be an impossible challenge. That's why parents and school staff should collaborate to find ways to accommodate children's academic and health needs. Here are some strategies parents can adopt:

· **Keep the lines of communication open.** Request a meeting with the school nurse, your child's teacher, and any appropriate administrators to explain what is going on with your child. Often, simply hearing about the ins and outs of your child's pain will help school staff understand the situation and be more inclined to allow for academic exceptions (such as extra time for homework, a reduced workload, or rescheduled tests).

· **Seek out an ally at school.** Having one point person at school (whether that's the school nurse, a guidance counselor, or a teacher) who knows what your child is going through can minimize complications and miscommunications. If your child needs to limit school attendance to half-days, for example, that point person becomes the one with whom you coordinate. When your child is on school grounds, that person can also be the staffer who keeps an eye out and serves as a resource if your child needs help.

· **Consider a 504 plan or an individualized education program (IEP).** Talk to your school administrators to see if your child qualifies for one of these federal designations, which were created to ensure that students with disabilities receive equal opportunities to learn and achieve. While the two programs have different origins (504 plans are specified by the Rehabilitation Act, and an IEP is part of the Individuals with Disabilities and Education Act), they are both meant for children whose disabilities (physical or cognitive) are affecting their school performance, and both laws generally offer individual accommodations, support, and / or services that help children learn to their fullest potential. A child with a 504 plan, for instance, may be given more time to finish homework assignments (say, if pain prohibits the child from typing for continued stretches), and a child with an IEP will often receive specialized instruction (say, a tutor at home or virtual lessons if the child is unable to go to school in person).

· **Be ready to advocate for your child.** Sometimes, even after explaining your child's situation to the school and developing a specialized plan, you may still encounter obstacles. In those cases, continue to be open with your child's teachers and administrators about the challenges you're facing, and if needed, talk with your child's healthcare practitioners and ask if they can either write notes or have conversations with school staff to help your child get the best possible accommodations for her condition. You may even want to enlist the help of a special education advocate familiar with the workings of the school system. Sometimes these advocates are volunteers within the community; in some cases they are education specialists who can be hired.

There are several ways to work toward these goals. Parents may encourage kids to pursue activities or interests, when possible. These might include cooking at home, joining an after-school club, or baby-sitting a neighbor's child. Taylor (from Chapter 9) keeps her CRPS at bay by horseback riding, which she adores. The activity keeps her ankle moving and gives her a sense of accomplishment. Adrian also remembers being determined in high school to become an athlete, an intellectual, and a guitar player. "I didn't want the sickle cell to define me," he says. "I wanted it to be a much smaller element of my life, so I was obsessed with defining who I was in other ways."

For many teenagers, finding a job in the community builds self-reliance and confidence, and teaches them they are valuable and needed. Having someone depend on them can also increase the chances they'll show up. One of Anna's patients with chronic leg pain had at one point stopped going to school in person and stopped participating in the youth group activities she liked because her pain had gotten worse. But she did not even think about stopping her job as the swim coach for a team of elementary school-aged kids three nights per week. When Anna asked her why she stuck with the swim team, she said, "Oh, I will *never* stop coaching swim. Those girls are counting on me."

Even in cases where kids don't have the energy, time, or ability to pursue an activity that might enhance their independence, parents can create opportunities for kids to gain autonomy by involving them directly in decisions about their healthcare. For younger children, parents can give kids choices about certain aspects of treatment, like which finger to prick for blood sugar tests (as Wendy did, in Chapter 5). For older children, parents might create space at medical appointments for kids to speak for themselves and share in decision-making about their care.

As grueling as it can be to manage chronic pain along with the stigma tied to it, parents are often astounded by the tenacity they see in their children. And the children, too, grow to recognize how strong they are. Some even seek out careers where they can share their healthcare knowledge and compassion. Emily now helps people manage invasive medical procedures in her job as a hospital social worker. Mina is training to be an occupational therapist. Adrian gives talks on wellness throughout his community. Tyler (from Chapter 9) plans to study medicine in college and become an orthopedic surgeon. Fiona (from Chapter 10) studied neuroscience in college on the pre-med track and hopes to be a physician's assistant.

"Even though I didn't want to be defined by concussions and chronic pain, I was really interested in learning how my brain was so resilient," says Fiona. "There were several times in high school when it looked so bleak—we really thought the reality was that I wouldn't graduate from high school. And forget about going to college! But when I was able to recover, I really wanted to know how my brain did it."

Stopping the Cycle

Preventing chronic pain in the next generation

It's amazing the reactions you get when you mention you're writing a book about children and pain. It's almost like a Rorschach test for what people think pain is. Some assume you must be talking about agonizing, rare conditions. Others immediately inform you that their child is "a wimp about pain" if he so much as stubs his toe. Occasionally, a person is quick to let you know that they don't believe in giving children opioids. Then, there are still other people who don't know quite what to say. "Pain in kids? What do you mean? Is that a big problem?" For all the misconceptions we have about pain, it seems we have even more about children and pain—namely, that kids don't get chronic pain, that children tend to fake their pain, and that temporary pain can't cause kids any lasting harm.

The problem with these fallacies is that they can cause both short-term and long-term damage. When adults don't recognize or adequately manage a child's pain, this not only hurts the child in that moment, it can also lay the foundation for a faulty pain response later on. Early pain that is poorly treated—whether it's due to a skinned knee, a needle prick, or an invasive surgery—can change a child's nervous system and lead to increased sensitivity to pain in the future, and a higher risk of chronic pain down the line.

Most people, and many medical professionals, are unaware of the ways that acute pain can affect children and are typically less aware of the effects—or even the existence—of chronic pain in children. Consequently, millions of children suffer unnecessarily with inadequate pain management, and up to two-thirds of the children who develop persistent pain grow into adults who have chronic pain. As adults, then, they typically face stigmatization and inadequate treatment for a disease many healthcare providers don't understand or believe is real.

This cycle can be stopped. We have the knowledge base, the tools, and the growing body of research to lessen kids' pain now and prevent it from becoming chronic. More than that, we have a moral and ethical obligation to do so.

The first steps? Increase education and raise awareness among parents, medical professionals, teachers, and other adults who care for children. Pain, often called the fifth vital sign, must be considered, evaluated, and managed from the first moments of a baby's life. How is it that there are parenting books devoted to nearly every aspect of caring for babies—how to help them sleep, nurse, eat, talk, read, behave, and so much more—yet there have been no books devoted to how to help babies through their first exposures to pain and the exposures that follow? Isn't the experience of pain as universally human as sleeping or eating? We argue, of course, that it is, and has been overlooked for too long.

We can change things for the next generation. We don't even need to look far off into the future to imagine it. What if all parents and pediatricians were aware of relaxation and distraction techniques that they could easily implement to reduce the intensity of a child's pain after a fall or during a vaccination? What if we all took notice when a child had her second or third headache, and could give her simple strategies that might prevent them from recurring and becoming disabling? What if a teenager confronting pain knew to pull out his smart phone or tablet to access a stress management app that could help him calm down and lessen the severity of his discomfort?

These possibilities are here now and they hold such promise to transform lives. We can see that promise, and we hope you can see it, too.

Helpful Resources

Websites on Children's Pain Management

American Academy of Pain Medicine
Resources for patients and clinicians
painmed.org

ChildKind
Offers a listing of ChildKind hospitals dedicated to improving pediatric pain care, and a resource library for clinicians and researchers
childkindinternational.org

The Comfort Ability
Offers nationwide workshops for families managing chronic pain; and apps and online resources
thecomfortability.com
thecomfortability.com/pages/apps-website-resources

It Doesn't Have to Hurt
Includes resources for parents, clinicians, and researchers
itdoesnthavetohurt.ca

Newborn Individualized Development Care and Assessment Program (NIDCAP)
Offers resources for families and clinicians caring for infants born prematurely
nidcap.org

Pain in Child Health (PICH)

A research training initiative in pediatric pain targeted at scientists and clinicians

paininchildhealth.ca

Special Interest Group on Pain in Childhood (Part of the International Association for the Study of Pain) Resource List

Includes an international directory of pediatric pain programs

childpain.org/index.php/resources

Solutions for Kids in Pain (SKIP)

A knowledge mobilization network that aims to bridge the gap between research and treatment practices

kidsinpain.ca

U.S. Pain Foundation

Offers resources on managing chronic pain

uspainfoundation.org

Books on How to Manage Children's Chronic Pain

Rachael Coakley, *When Your Child Hurts: Effective Strategies to Increase Comfort, Reduce Stress, and Break the Cycle of Chronic Pain* (New Haven, CT: Yale University Press, 2016)

Elliot J. Krane with Deborah Mitchell, *Relieve Your Child's Chronic Pain: A Doctor's Program for Easing Headaches, Abdominal Pain, Fibromyalgia, Juvenile Rheumatoid Arthritis, and More* (New York: Simon & Schuster, 2005)

Tonya M. Palermo and Emily F. Law, *Managing Your Child's Chronic Pain* (New York: Oxford University Press, 2015)

Lonnie K. Zeltzer and Christina Blackett Schlank, *Conquering Your Child's Chronic Pain: A Pediatrician's Guide for Reclaiming a Normal Childhood* (New York: HarperCollins, 2005)

Notes

Introduction

1. J. Dahlhamer, J. Lucas, C. Zelaya, et al., "Prevalence of Chronic Pain and High-Impact Chronic Pain among Adults—United States, 2016," *Morbidity and Mortality Weekly Report* 67, no. 36 (2018): 1001; D. J. Gaskin and P. Richard, "The Economic Costs of Pain in the United States," *Journal of Pain* 13, no. 8 (2012): 715–724; L. S. Simon, "Relieving Pain in America: A Blueprint for Transforming Prevention, Care, Education, and Research," *Journal of Pain and Palliative Care Pharmacotherapy* 26, no. 2 (2012): 197–198.

2. US Department of Health and Human Services, "What Is the U.S. Opioid Epidemic?" October 27, 2021, https://www.hhs.gov/opioids/about-the-epidemic/index.html.

3. C. B. Groenewald, B. S. Essner, D. Wright, M. D. Fesinmeyer, and T. M. Palermo, "The Economic Costs of Chronic Pain among a Cohort of Treatment-Seeking Adolescents in the United States," *Journal of Pain* 15, no. 9 (2014): 925–933; A. Huguet and J. Miró, "The Severity of Chronic Pediatric Pain: An Epidemiological Study," *Journal of Pain* 9, no. 3 (2008): 226–236; S. King, C. T. Chambers, A. Huguet, et al., "The Epidemiology of Chronic Pain in Children and Adolescents Revisited: A Systematic Review," *Pain* 152, no. 12 (2011): 2729–2738.

4. E. V. Briggs, E. C. J. Carr, and M. S. Whittaker, "Survey of Undergraduate Pain Curricula for Healthcare Professionals in the United Kingdom," *European Journal of Pain* 15, no. 8 (2011): 789–795; L. Mezei and B. B. Murinson, "Pain Education in North American Medical Schools," *Journal of Pain* 12, no. 12 (2011): 1199–1208; J. Watt-Watson, M. McGillion, J. Hunter, et al., "A Survey of Prelicensure Pain Curricula in Health Science Faculties in Canadian Universities," *Pain Research and Management* 14, no. 6 (2009): 439–444.
5. King et al., "Epidemiology of Chronic Pain"; L. E. Simons, D. E. Logan, L. Chastain, and M. Cerullo, "Engagement in Multidisciplinary Interventions for Pediatric Chronic Pain: Parental Expectations, Barriers, and Child Outcomes," *Clinical Journal of Pain* 26, no. 4 (2010): 291–299; E. A. Stanford, C. T. Chambers, J. C. Biesanz, and E. Chen, "The Frequency, Trajectories and Predictors of Adolescent Recurrent Pain: A Population-Based Approach," *Pain* 138, no. 1 (2008): 11–21.
6. Simons et al., "Engagement in Multidisciplinary Interventions."
7. A. Lloyd-Thomas, "Pain Management in Paediatric Patients," *British Journal of Anaesthesia* 64, no. 1 (1990): 85–104.
8. A. Taddio, J. Katz, A. L. Ilersich, and G. Koren, "Effect of Neonatal Circumcision on Pain Response during Subsequent Routine Vaccination," *Lancet* 349, no. 9052 (1997): 599–603.
9. A. Oxman and S. Flottorp, "An Overview of Strategies to Promote Implementation of Evidence-Based Health Care," *Evidence-Based Practice in Primary Care* 2 (2001): 101–119.

Chapter 1: How and Why Do We Feel Pain?

1. A. Benini and J. A. DeLeo, "René Descartes' Physiology of Pain," *Spine* 24, no. 20 (1999): 2115–2119; L. A. Trachsel and M. Cascella, "Pain Theory," *StatPearls* (Internet), updated August 2, 2021, https://www.ncbi.nlm.nih.gov/books/NBK545194/.
2. S. N. Raja, D. B. Carr, M. Cohen, et al., "The Revised International Association for the Study of Pain Definition of Pain: Concepts, Challenges, and Compromises," *Pain* 161, no. 9 (2020): 1976–1982.

3. R. Melzack, interview by Leora Kuttner, for documentary "Children in Pain," April 1989, https://www.youtube.com/watch?v=0qGZPmUttUk.

4. N. Ahimsadasan, V. Reddy, and A. Kumar, "Neuroanatomy, Dorsal Root Ganglion," *StatPearls* (Internet), updated September 7, 2021, https://pubmed.ncbi.nlm.nih.gov/30335324/; M. Devor, "Obituary: Patrick David Wall, 1925–2001," *Pain* 94, no. 2 (2001): 125–129.

5. G. Lorimer Moseley, *Painful Yarns: Metaphors and Stories to Help Understand the Biology of Pain* (Minneapolis: Orthopedic Physical Therapy Products, 2007).

6. Moseley, *Painful Yarns*.

7. S. King, C. T. Chambers, A. Huguet, et al., "The Epidemiology of Chronic Pain in Children and Adolescents Revisited: A Systematic Review," *Pain* 152, no. 12 (2011): 2729–2738.

8. R. C. B. Manworren and J. Stinson, "Pediatric Pain Measurement, Assessment, and Evaluation. *Seminars in Pediatric Neurology* 23, no. 3 (2016): 189–200.

9. C. T. Chambers and J. S. Mogil, "Ontogeny and Phylogeny of Facial Expression of Pain," *Pain* 156, no. 5 (2015): 798–799.

10. Manworren and Stinson, "Pediatric Pain Measurement"; 12. L. K. Murphy, R. de la Vega, S. A. Kohut, J. S. Kawamura, R. L. Levy, and T. M. Palermo, "Systematic Review: Psychosocial Correlates of Pain in Pediatric Inflammatory Bowel Disease," *Inflammatory Bowel Diseases* 27, no. 5 (2021): 697–910; C. V. Bellieni, R. Sisto, D. M. Cordelli, and G. Buonocore, "Cry Features Reflect Pain Intensity in Term Newborns: An Alarm Threshold," *Pediatric Research* 55, no. 1 (2004): 142–146; A. Koutseff, D. Reby, O. Martin, F. Levrero, H. Patural, and N. Mathevon, "The Acoustic Space of Pain: Cries as Indicators of Distress Recovering Dynamics in Pre-verbal Infants," *Bioacoustics* 27, no. 4 (2018): 313–325; T. Naik, A. Thommandram, K. E. S. Fernando, N. Bressan, A. James, and C. A. McGregor, "Method for a Real-Time Novel Premature Infant Pain Profile Using High Rate, High Volume Physiological Data Streams," paper presented at IEEE 27th International Symposium on Computer-Based Medical Systems, May 27–29, 2014; M. Schiavenato and C. L. von Baeyer, "A Quantitative Examination of Extreme Facial Pain Expression in Neonates: The Primal Face of Pain across Time," *Pain Research and Treatment* (2012): art. 251625.

11. A. Lewandowski Holley, J. Rabbitts, C. Zhou, L. Durkin, and
     T. M. Palermo, "Temporal Daily Associations among Sleep and Pain
     in Treatment-Seeking Youth with Acute Musculoskeletal Pain,"
     Journal of Behavioral Medicine 40, no. 4 (2017): 675–681.
12. Manworren and Stinson, "Pediatric Pain Measurement"; T. M. Palermo,
     D. Valenzuela, and P. P. Stork, "A Randomized Trial of Electronic
     versus Paper Pain Diaries in Children: Impact on Compliance,
     Accuracy, and Acceptability," *Pain* 107, no. 3 (2004): 213–219;
     J. N. Stinson, L. A. Jibb, C. Nguyen, et al., "Construct Validity and
     Reliability of a Real-Time Multidimensional Smartphone App to
     Assess Pain in Children and Adolescents with Cancer," *Pain* 156,
     no. 12 (2015): 2607–2615.
13. S. Mulvaney, E. W. Lambert, J. Garber, and L. S. Walker, "Trajectories
     of Symptoms and Impairment for Pediatric Patients with Functional
     Abdominal Pain: A 5-Year Longitudinal Study," *Journal of the
     American Academy of Child and Adolescent Psychiatry* 45, no. 6
     (2006): 737–744.

Chapter 2: Little Kids Won't Remember It Anyway, Right?

1. N. C. Butler, "How to Raise Professional Awareness of the Need for
    Adequate Pain Relief for Infants," *Birth* 15, no. 1 (1988): 38–41;
    J. R. Lawson, Letter, *Birth* 13, no. 2 (1986): 124–125.
2. A. M. Unruh and P. J. McGrath, *History of Pain in Children*
    (Oxford: Oxford University Press, 2014).
3. N. C. Butler, "Infants, Pain, and What Health Care Professionals
    Should Want to Know—An Issue of Epistemology and Ethics," *Bioethics*
    3, no. 3 (1989): 181–199; R. Gustaitis and E. W. Young, *A Time to
    Be Born, a Time to Die: Conflicts and Ethics in an Intensive Care
    Nursery* (Reading, MA: Addison-Wesley, 1986).
4. E. T. Boie, G. P. Moore, C. Brummett, and D. R. Nelson, "Do Parents
    Want to Be Present during Invasive Procedures Performed on Their
    Children in the Emergency Department? A Survey of 400 Parents,"
    Annals of Emergency Medicine 34, no. 1 (1999): 70–74; K. A. Merritt,
    P. A. Ornstein, and B. Spicker, "Children's Memory for a Salient
    Medical Procedure: Implications for Testimony," *Pediatrics* 94, no. 1
    (1994): 17–23.

5. E. N. Rodkey and R. Pillai Riddell, "The Infancy of Infant Pain Research: The Experimental Origins of Infant Pain Denial," *Journal of Pain* 14, no. 4 (2013): 338–350.

6. P. J. McGrath and A. M. Unruh, *Pain in Children and Adolescents* (New York: Elsevier, 1987).

7. Hippocrates, "On the Sacred Disease," in T. M. Walshe, *Neurological Concepts in Ancient Greek Medicine* (Oxford: Oxford University Press, 2016).

8. C. F. Kleisiaris, C. Sfakianakis, and I. V. Papathanasiou, "Health Care Practices in Ancient Greece: The Hippocratic Ideal," *Journal of Medical Ethics and History of Medicine* 7 (2014): 6.

9. Galen, *Hygiene (De Sanitate Tuenda)*, ed. and trans. Ian Johnston, Loeb Classical Library 535 (Cambridge, MA: Harvard University Press, 2018), Book one, chapter 7. See also G. F. Still, *The History of Paediatrics: The Progress of the Study of Diseases of Children up to the End of the XVIIIth Century* (London: Oxford University Press, 1931), 32–33.

10. Plutarch, "Lycurgus," *Plutarch's Lives, Volume One*, trans. John Dryden (New York: Modern Library, 2001), 67. Also see F. H. Garrison, *A System of Pediatrics, Vol. 1* (Philadelphia, PA: Saunders, 1923): 1–61, quote on 35.

11. J. B. Watson, *Psychological Care of Infant and Child* (New York: W. W. Norton, 1928).

12. S. Smiles, *Physical Education; or, the Nurture and Management of Children, Founded on the Study of Their Nature and Constitution* (London: Oliver and Boyd, 1838).

13. L. Starr, "The Clinical Investigation of Disease and the General Management of Children," in *An American Text-book of the Diseases of Children* ed. L. Starr, 1–36 (Philadelphia: W. B. Saunders, 1895).

14. T. B. Brazelton, *To Listen to a Child: Understanding the Normal Problems of Growing Up* (Reading, MA: Addison-Wesley, 1984); T. B. Brazelton and J. K. Nugent, *Neonatal Behavioral Assessment Scale* (Cambridge: Cambridge University Press, 1995); B. Spock, *The Common Sense Book of Baby and Child Care* (New York: Duell, Sloan and Pearce, 1946).

15. R. Fülöp-Miller, *Triumph over Pain* (New York: Literary Guild of America, 1938).

16. Lawson, letter; L. Caes, K. E. Boerner, C. T. Chambers, et al., "A Comprehensive Categorical and Bibliometric Analysis of Published Research Articles on Pediatric Pain from 1975 to 2010," *Pain* 157, no. 2 (2016): 302–313; E. Guardiola and J.-E. Baños, "Is There an Increasing Interest in Pediatric Pain? Analysis of the Biomedical Articles Published in the 1980s," *Journal of Pain and Symptom Management* 8, no. 7 (1993): 449–450; P. J. McGrath, "Science Is Not Enough: The Modern History of Pediatric Pain," *Pain* 152, no. 11 (2011): 2457–2459.

17. S. Rovner, "Surgery without Anesthesia: Can Preemies Feel Pain?" *Washington Post,* August 13, 1986.

18. American Academy of Pediatrics, "Neonatal Anesthesia," *Pediatrics* 80, no. 3 (1987): 446; P. R. Tutelman and C. T. Chambers, "Moving from Knowledge to Action in Pediatric Pain: A Look at the Past, Present and Future," *Pediatric Pain Letter* 18, no. 3 (2016): 22–25.

19. A. B. Fletcher, "Pain in the Neonate," *New England Journal of Medicine* 317, no. 21 (1987): 1347–1348.

20. K. J. S. Anand, M. J. Brown, S. R. Bloom, and A. Aynsley-Green, "Studies on the Hormonal Regulation of Fuel Metabolism in the Human Newborn Infant Undergoing Anaesthesia and Surgery," *Hormone Research in Paediatrics* 22, no. 1–2 (1985): 115–128.

21. K. J. S. Anand, W. G. Sippell, and A. Aynsley-Green, "Randomised Trial of Fentanyl Anaesthesia in Preterm Babies Undergoing Surgery: Effects on the Stress Response," *Lancet* 329, no. 8527 (1987): 243–248.

22. K. J. S. Anand and P. R. Hickey, "Pain and Its Effects in the Human Neonate and Fetus," *New England Journal of Medicine* 317, no. 21 (1987): 1321–1329.

23. K. J. S. Anand, D. D. Hansen, and P. R. Hickey, "Hormonal-Metabolic Stress Responses in Neonates Undergoing Cardiac Surgery," *Anesthesiology* 73, no. 4 (1990): 661–670; K. J. S. Anand and P. R. Hickey, "Halothane-Morphine Compared with High-Dose Sufentanil for Anesthesia and Postoperative Analgesia in Neonatal Cardiac Surgery," *New England Journal of Medicine* 326, no. 1 (1992): 1–9.

24. H. N. Turner, "Jo Eland May Be Gone, but Her Legacy Remains," *Pain Management Nursing* 17, no. 6 (2016): 352–353.

25. J. E. Beyer, "Judging the Effectiveness of Analgesia for Children and Adolescents during Vaso-occlusive Events of Sickle Cell Disease," *Journal of Pain Symptom Management* 19, no. 1 (2000): 63–72; C. Knott, J. Beyer, A. Villarruel, M. Denyes, V. Erickson, and G. Willard, "Developmental Approach to Pain Assessment in Children: How, Why, and When to Use the Original Oucher and Two New Ethnic Versions," *MCN: The American Journal of Maternal/Child Nursing* 19, no. 6 (1994): 314–320; J. E. Beyer and C. R. Aradine, "Patterns of Pediatric Pain Intensity: A Methodological Investigation of a Self-Report Scale," *Clinical Journal of Pain* 3, no. 3 (1987): 130–141; J. Beyer, *The Oucher: A User's Manual and Technical Report* (Evanston, IL: The Hospital Play Equipment Company, 1984).

26. N. L. Schechter, D. A. Allen, amd K. Hanson, "Status of Pediatric Pain Control: A Comparison of Hospital Analgesic Usage in Children and Adults," *Pediatrics* 77, no. 1 (1986): 11–15.

27. N. L. Schechter, "The Undertreatment of Pain in Children: An Overview," *Pediatric Clinics of North America* 36, no. 4 (1989): 781–794; N. L. Schechter and D. Allen, "Physicians' Attitudes toward Pain in Children," *Journal of Developmental and Behavioral Pediatrics* 7, no. 6 (1986): 350–354.

28. G. A. Finley and P. J. McGrath, eds., *Measurement of Pain in Infants and Children* (Seattle: IASP Press, 1998).

29. C. L. von Baeyer, B. J. Stevens, K. D. Craig, et al., "Pain in Child Health from 2002 to 2015: The Early Years of an International Research Training Initiative," *Canadian Journal of Pain* 3, no. 1 (2019): 1–7.

30. A. Oxman and S. Flottorp, "An Overview of Strategies to Promote Implementation of Evidence-Based Health Care," in *Evidence-Based Practice in Primary Care,* 2nd ed., ed. C. Silagy and A. Haines (London: BMJ Press, 2001), 101–119.

31. J. Watt-Watson, M. McGillion, J. Hunter, et al., A Survey of Prelicensure Pain Curricula in Health Science Faculties in Canadian Universities," *Pain Research and Management* 14, no. 6 (2009): 439–444.

32. For more information on SKIP, see the program website: https://kids inpain.ca/.

33. T. M. Palermo, M. Slack, C. Zhou, R. Aaron, E. Fisher, and S. Rodriguez, "Waiting for a Pediatric Chronic Pain Clinic Evaluation: A Prospective

Study Characterizing Waiting Times and Symptom Trajectories," *Journal of Pain* 20, no. 3 (2019): 339–347; P. Peng, J. N. Stinson, M. Choiniere, et al., "Dedicated Multidisciplinary Pain Management Centres for Children in Canada: The Current Status," *Canadian Journal of Anaesthesiology* 54, no. 12 (2007): 985–991.

Chapter 3: Ouch!

1. D. Harrison, C. Larocque, M. Bueno, et al., "Sweet Solutions to Reduce Procedural Pain in Neonates: A Meta-analysis," *Pediatrics* 139, no. 1 (2017), e20160955; D. Harrison, J. Reszel, M. Bueno, et al., "Breastfeeding for Procedural Pain in Infants beyond the Neonatal Period," *Cochrane Database of Systematic Reviews* update, October 28, 2016, CD011248; C. McNair, M. Campbell-Yeo, C. Johnston, and A. Taddio, "Nonpharmacologic Management of Pain during Common Needle Puncture Procedures in Infants: Current Research Evidence and Practical Considerations: An Update," *Clinics in Perinatology* 46, no. 4 (2019): 709–730; A. Taddio, C. M. McMurtry, V. Shah, et al., "Reducing Pain during Vaccine Injections: Clinical Practice Guideline," *Canadian Medical Association Journal* 187, no. 13 (2015): 975–982.

2. C. M. McMurtry, R. Pillai Riddell, A. Taddio, et al., "Far from "Just a Poke": Common Painful Needle Procedures and the Development of Needle Fear," *Clinical Journal of Pain* 31, no. 10 suppl. (2015): S3–S11.

3. V. Ianelli, "Vaccines Statistics and Numbers," *Vaxopedia* (V. Ianelli), March 4, 2020, https://vaxopedia.org/2018/01/10/vaccines-statistics -and-numbers/.

4. B. Deacon and J. Abramowitz, "Fear of Needles and Vasovagal Reactions among Phlebotomy Patients," *Journal of Anxiety Disorders* 20, no. 7 (2006): 946–960; A. Taddio, M. Ipp, S. Thivakaran, et al., "Survey of the Prevalence of Immunization Non-compliance Due to Needle Fears in Children and Adults," *Vaccine* 30, no. 32 (2012): 4807–4812.

5. American Academy of Pediatrics, "Prevention and Management of Procedural Pain in the Neonate: An Update," *Pediatrics* 137, no. 2 (2016), e20154271.

6. M. L. Campbell-Yeo, T. C. Disher, B. L. Benoit, and C. C. Johnston, "Understanding Kangaroo Care and Its Benefits to Preterm Infants," *Pediatric Health Medicine and Therapeutics* 6 (2015): 15–32.

7. D. Harrison, J. Wilding, A. Bowman, et al., "Using YouTube to Disseminate Effective Vaccination Pain Treatment for Babies," *PLoS One* 11, no. 10 (2016), e0164123; D. Harrison, J. Yamada, T. Adams-Webber, A. Ohlsson, J. Beyene, and B. Stevens, "Sweet Tasting Solutions for Reduction of Needle-Related Procedural Pain in Children Aged One to 16 Years," *Cochrane Database of Systematic Reviews,* May 5, 2015, CD008408.

8. K. A. Birnie, C. T. Chambers, A. Taddio, et al., "Psychological Interventions for Vaccine Injections in Children and Adolescents: Systematic Review of Randomized and Quasi-Randomized Controlled Trials," *Clinical Journal of Pain* 31, no. 10 suppl. (2015): S72–S89.

9. K. A. Birnie, M. Noel, J. A. Parker, et al., "Systematic Review and Meta-analysis of Distraction and Hypnosis for Needle-Related Pain and Distress in Children and Adolescents," *Journal of Pediatric Psychology* 39, no. 8 (2014): 783–808.

10. V. Shah, A. Taddio, C. M. McMurtry, et al., "Pharmacological and Combined Interventions to Reduce Vaccine Injection Pain in Children and Adults: Systematic Review and Meta-analysis," *Clinical Journal of Pain* 31, no. 10 suppl. (2015): S38–S63.

11. L. L. Cohen, R. L. Blount, R. J. Cohen, E. R. Schaen, and J. F. Zaff, "Comparative Study of Distraction versus Topical Anesthesia for Pediatric Pain Management during Immunizations," *Health Psychology* 18, no. 6 (1999): 591–598.

12. L. L. Cohen, J. E. MacLaren, B. L. Fortson, et al., "Randomized Clinical Trial of Distraction for Infant Immunization Pain," *Pain* 125, no. 1 (2006): 165–171.

13. M. Noel, C. T. Chambers, P. J. McGrath, R. M. Klein, and S. H. Stewart, "The Influence of Children's Pain Memories on Subsequent Pain Experience," *Pain* 153, no. 8 (2012): 1563–1572.

14. T. A. Marche, J. L. Briere, and C. L. von Baeyer, "Children's Forgetting of Pain-Related Memories," *Journal of Pediatric Psychology* 41, no. 2 (2016): 220–231; M. Noel, C. M. McMurtry, C. T. Chambers, and P. J. McGrath, "Children's Memory for Painful Procedures: The Relationship of Pain Intensity, Anxiety, and Adult Behaviors to

Subsequent Recall," *Journal of Pediatric Psychology* 35, no. 6 (2009): 626–636.

15. S. Badovinac, H. Gennis, R. P. Riddell, H. Garfield, and S. Greenberg, "Understanding the Relative Contributions of Sensitive and Insensitive Parent Behaviors on Infant Vaccination Pain," *Children* 5, no. 6 (2018): 80; L. Campbell, R. Pillai Riddell, R. Cribbie, H. Garfield, and S. Greenberg, "Preschool Children's Coping Responses and Outcomes in the Vaccination Context: Child and Caregiver Transactional and Longitudinal Relationships," *Pain* 159, no. 2 (2018): 314–330; N. M. Racine, R. R. Pillai Riddell, D. B. Flora, A. Taddio, H. Garfield, and S. Greenberg, "Predicting Preschool Pain-Related Anticipatory Distress: The Relative Contribution of Longitudinal and Concurrent Factors," *Pain* 157, no. 9 (2016): 1918–1932.

16. C. M. McMurtry, C. T. Chambers, P. J. McGrath, and E. Asp, "When 'Don't Worry' Communicates Fear: Children's Perceptions of Parental Reassurance and Distraction during a Painful Medical Procedure," *Pain* 150, no. 1 (2010): 52–58.

17. A. Oxman and S. Flottorp, "An Overview of Strategies to Promote Implementation of Evidence-Based Health Care," *Evidence-Based Practice in Primary Care* 2 (2001): 101–119.

18. S. J. Friedrichsdorf and L. Goubert, "Pediatric Pain Treatment and Prevention for Hospitalized Children," *Pain Reports* 5, no. 1 (2020), e804.

Chapter 4: Scars from the NICU

1. R. Carbajal, A. Rousset, C. Danan, et al., "Epidemiology and Treatment of Painful Procedures in Neonates in Intensive Care Units," *JAMA* 300, no. 1 (2008): 60–70.

2. J. Vinall, S. P. Miller, B. H. Bjornson, et al., "Invasive Procedures in Preterm Children: Brain and Cognitive Development at School Age," *Pediatrics* 133, no. 3 (2014): 412–421.

3. S. Brummelte, R. E. Grunau, V. Chau, et al., "Procedural Pain and Brain Development in Premature Newborns," *Annals of Neurology* 71, no. 3 (2012): 385–396; M. Ranger and R. E. Grunau, "Early Repetitive Pain in Preterm Infants in Relation to the Developing Brain," *Pain Management* 4, no. 1 (2014): 57–67.

4. K. Anand and F. M. Scalzo, "Can Adverse Neonatal Experiences Alter Brain Development and Subsequent Behavior?" *Neonatology* 77, no. 2 (2000): 69–82; M. Fitzgerald, "What Do We Really Know about Newborn Infant Pain?" *Experimental Physiology* 100, no. 12 (2015): 1451–1457; C. C. Johnston, A. M. Fernandes, and M. Campbell-Yeo, "Pain in Neonates Is Different," *Pain* 152, no. 3 suppl. (2011): S65–S73; N. J. van den Hoogen, J. Patijn, D. Tibboel, B. A. Joosten, M. Fitzgerald, and C. H. T. Kwok, "Repeated Touch and Needle-Prick Stimulation in the Neonatal Period Increases the Baseline Mechanical Sensitivity and Postinjury Hypersensitivity of Adult Spinal Sensory Neurons," *Pain* 159, no. 6 (2018): 1166–1175.

5. K. Anand, "Prevention and Treatment of Neonatal Pain," UpToDate, updated May 28, 2021.

6. R. E. Grunau, "Early Pain in Preterm Infants: A Model of Long-Term Effects," *Clinics in Perinatology* 29, no. 3 (2002): 373–394.

7. L. Fabrizi, R. Slater, A. Worley, et al., "A Shift in Sensory Processing That Enables the Developing Human Brain to Discriminate Touch from Pain," *Current Biology* 21, no. 18 (2011): 1552–1558; R. Slater, L. Fabrizi, A. Worley, J. Meek, S. Boyd, and M. Fitzgerald, "Premature Infants Display Increased Noxious-Evoked Neuronal Activity in the Brain Compared to Healthy Age-Matched Term-Born Infants," *Neuroimage* 52, no. 2 (2010): 583–589.

8. S. Goksan, L. Baxter, F. Moultrie, et al., "The Influence of the Descending Pain Modulatory System on Infant Pain-Related Brain Activity," *eLife* 7 (2018), e37125.

9. R. V. Grunau, C. C. Johnston, and K. D. Craig, "Neonatal Facial and Cry Responses to Invasive and Non-invasive Procedures," *Pain* 42, no. 3 (1990): 295–305; R. V. E. Grunau, "Cry and Facial Behavior during Induced Pain in Neonates" (PhD diss., University of British Columbia, 1985); C. C. Johnston and M. E. Strada, "Acute Pain Response in Infants: A Multidimensional Description," *Pain* 24, no. 3 (1986): 373–382.

10. F. Schwaller and M. Fitzgerald, "The Consequences of Pain in Early Life: Injury-Induced Plasticity in Developing Pain Pathways," *European Journal of Neuroscience* 39, no. 3 (2014): 344–352; S. M. Walker, S. Beggs and M. L. Baccei, "Persistent Changes in Peripheral and

Spinal Nociceptive Processing after Early Tissue Injury," *Experimental Neurology* 275 (2016): 253–260.

11. C. Johnston, M. Campbell-Yeo, T. Disher, et al., "Skin-to-Skin Care for Procedural Pain in Neonates," *Cochrane Database of Systematic Reviews,* February 16, 2017, CD008435.

12. M. Campbell-Yeo, C. C. Johnston, B. Benoit, et al., "Sustained Efficacy of Kangaroo Care for Repeated Painful Procedures over Neonatal Intensive Care Unit Hospitalization: A Single-Blind Randomized Controlled Trial," *Pain* 160, no. 11 (2019): 2580–2588; M. L. Campbell-Yeo, T. C. Disher, B. L. Benoit, and C. C. Johnston, "Understanding Kangaroo Care and Its Benefits to Preterm Infants," *Pediatric Health, Medicine and Therapeutics* 6 (2015): 15–32.

13. D. Harrison, S. Beggs, and B. Stevens, "Sucrose for Procedural Pain Management in Infants," *Pediatrics* 130, no. 5 (2012): 918–925; D. Harrison, C. Larocque, M. Bueno, et al., "Sweet Solutions to Reduce Procedural Pain in Neonates: A Meta-analysis," *Pediatrics* 139, no. 1 (2017), e20160955.

14. M. Ranger, S. Tremblay, C. M. Chau, L. Holsti, R. E. Grunau, and D. Goldowitz, "Adverse Behavioral Changes in Adult Mice Following Neonatal Repeated Exposure to Pain and Sucrose," *Frontiers in Psychology* 9 (2019), article 2394; S. Tremblay, M. Ranger, C. M. Chau, et al., "Repeated Exposure to Sucrose for Procedural Pain in Mouse Pups Leads to Long-Term Widespread Brain Alterations," *Pain* 158, no. 8 (2017): 1586–1598.

15. S. Hauser, M. J. Suto, L. Holsti, M. Ranger, and K. E. MacLean, "Designing and Evaluating Calmer, a Device for Simulating Maternal Skin-to-Skin Holding for Premature Infants," in Proceedings of the 2020 CHI Conference on Human Factors in Computing Systems, Honolulu, HI, April 2020, https://dl.acm.org/doi/pdf/10.1145/3313831.3376539; L. Holsti, K. E. MacLean, T. F. Oberlander, A. R. Synnes, and R. Brant, "Calmer: A Robot for Managing Acute Pain Effectively in Preterm Infants in the Neonatal Intensive Care Unit," *Pain Reports* 4, no. 2 (2019), e727.

16. H. Als and T. B. Brazelton, "A New Model of Assessing the Behavioral Organization in Preterm and Fullterm Infants: Two Case Studies," *Journal of the American Academy of Child Psychiatry* 20,

no. 2 (1981): 239–263; H. Als and G. B. McAnulty, "The Newborn Individualized Developmental Care and Assessment Program (NIDCAP) with Kangaroo Mother Care (KMC): Comprehensive Care for Preterm Infants. *Current Women's Health Reviews* 7, no. 3 (2011): 288–301.

17. G. P. Aylward, "Neurodevelopmental Outcomes of Infants Born Prematurely," *Journal of Developmental and Behavioral Pediatrics* 35, no. 6 (2014): 394–407; S. A. Reijneveld, M. J. K. de Kleine, A. L. van Baar, et al., "Behavioural and Emotional Problems in Very Preterm and Very Low Birthweight Infants at Age 5 Years," *Archives of Disease in Childhood—Fetal and Neonatal Edition* 91, no. 6 (2006): F423–F428; K. Schadl, R. Vassar, K. Cahill-Rowley, K. W. Yeom, D. K. Stevenson, and J. Rose, "Prediction of Cognitive and Motor Development in Preterm Children Using Exhaustive Feature Selection and Cross-Validation of Near-Term White Matter Microstructure," *NeuroImage: Clinical* 17 (2018): 667–679; L. T. Singer, A. C. Siegel, B. Lewis, S. Hawkins, T. Yamashita, and J. Baley, "Preschool Language Outcomes of Children with History of Bronchopulmonary Dysplasia and Very Low Birth Weight," *Journal of Developmental and Behavioral Pediatrics* 22, no. 1 (2001): 19–26.

18. A. Taddio, J. Katz, A. L. Ilersich, and G. Koren, "Effect of Neonatal Circumcision on Pain Response during Subsequent Routine Vaccination," *Lancet* 349, no. 9052 (1997): 599–603.

19. M. Bueno, B. Stevens, M. A. Barwick, et al., "A Cluster Randomized Clinical Trial to Evaluate the Effectiveness of the Implementation of Infant Pain Practice Change (ImPaC) Resource to Improve Pain Practices in Hospitalized Infants: A Study Protocol," *Trials* 21, no. 1 (2020), article 16.

20. M. Campbell-Yeo, A. Fernandes, and C. Johnston, "Procedural Pain Management for Neonates Using Nonpharmacological Strategies: Part 2: Mother-Driven Interventions," *Advances in Neonatal Care* 11, no. 5 (2011): 312–318.

21. C. McNair, M. Campbell-Yeo, C. Johnston, and A. Taddio, "Nonpharmacological Management of Pain during Common Needle Puncture Procedures in Infants: Current Research Evidence and Practical Considerations: An Update," *Clinics in Perinatology* 46 no. 4 (2019): 709–730.

Chapter 5: Surgeries, Minor Medical Procedures, and Hospital Visits

1.   J. A. Rabbitts, C. B. Groenewald, J. P. Moriarty, and R. Flick, "Epidemiology of Ambulatory Anesthesia for Children in the United States: 2006 and 1996," *Anesthesia and Analgesia* 111, no. 4 (2000): 1011–1015; K. Y. Tzong, S. Han, A. Roh, and C. Ing, "Epidemiology of Pediatric Surgical Admissions in US Children: Data from the HCUP Kids Inpatient Database," *Journal of Neurosurgical Anesthesiology* 24, no. 4 (2012): 391–395.

2.   National Institute for Health and Care Excellence (UK), "Sedation in Under 19s: Using Sedation for Diagnostic and Therapeutic Procedures, Clinical Guideline," Clinical Guideline 112, December 15, 2010, https://www.nice.org.uk/guidance/cg112/chapter/Introduction; M. Zielinska, A. Bartkowska-Sniatkowska, K. Becke, et al., "Safe Pediatric Procedural Sedation and Analgesia by Anesthesiologists for Elective Procedures: A Clinical Practice Statement from the European Society for Paediatric Anaesthesiology," *Pediatric Anesthesia* 29, no. 6 (2019): 583–590.

3.   Massachusetts General Hospital, "You Are Here: Wendy's Welcome to the ED," MGH for Children, Emergency Department, n.d., https://www.massgeneral.org/children/emergency-medicine/you-are -here-wendys-welcome-to-the-ed.

4.   A. Yahya Al-Sagarat, H. M. Al-Oran, H. Obeidat, A. M. Hamlan, and L. Moxham, "Preparing the Family and Children for Surgery," *Critical Care Nursing Quarterly* 40, no. 2 (2017): 99–107.

5.   Z. N. Kain, L. C. Mayes, A. A. Caldwell-Andrews, D. E. Karas, and B. C. McClain, "Preoperative Anxiety, Postoperative Pain, and Behavioral Recovery in Young Children Undergoing Surgery," *Pediatrics* 118, no. 2 (2006): 651–658; L. L. Lamontagne, J. T. Hepworth, and M. H. Salisbury, "Anxiety and Postoperative Pain in Children Who Undergo Major Orthopedic Surgery," *Applied Nursing Research* 14, no. 3 (2001): 119–124.

6.   H. Kim, S. M. Jung, H. Yu, and S. J. Park, "Video Distraction and Parental Presence for the Management of Preoperative Anxiety and Postoperative Behavioral Disturbance in Children: A Randomized Controlled Trial," *Anesthesia and Analgesia* 121, no. 3 (2015): 778–784; A. Manyande, A. M. Cyna, P. Yip, C. Chooi, and P. Middleton, "Non-pharmacological Interventions for Assisting the

Induction of Anaesthesia in Children," *Cochrane Database Systematic Reviews,* July 14, 2015, CD006447; A. Patel, T. Schieble, M. Davidson, et al., "Distraction with a Hand-Held Video Game Reduces Pediatric Preoperative Anxiety," *Paediatric Anaesthesia* 16, no. 10 (2006): 1019–1027.

7. S. Calipel, M. M. Lucas-Polomeni, E. Wodey, and C. Ecoffey, "Premedication in Children: Hypnosis versus Midazolam," *Paediatric Anaesthesia* 15, no. 4 (2005): 275–281.

8. L. Vagnoli, A. Bettini, E. Amore, S. De Masi, and A. Messeri, "Relaxation-Guided Imagery Reduces Perioperative Anxiety and Pain in Children: A Randomized Study," *European Journal of Pediatrics* 178, no. 6 (2019): 913–921.

9. Z. N. Kain, S.-M. Wang, L. C. Mayes, D. M. Krivutza, and B. A. Teague, "Sensory Stimuli and Anxiety in Children Undergoing Surgery: A Randomized, Controlled Trial," *Anesthesia and Analgesia* 92, no. 4 (2001): 897–903.

10. Z. N. Kain, L. C. Mayes, L. A. Caramico, et al., "Parental Presence during Induction of Anesthesia: A Randomized Controlled Trial," *Anesthesiology* 84, no. 5 (1996): 1060–1067.

11. N. L. Schechter, S. J. Weisman, M. Rosenblum, B. Bernstein, and P. L. Conard, "The Use of Oral Transmucosal Fentanyl Citrate for Painful Procedures in Children," *Pediatrics* 95, no. 3 (1995): 335–339; S. J. Weisman, B. Bernstein, and N. L. Schechter, "Consequences of Inadequate Analgesia during Painful Procedures in Children," *Archives of Pediatrics and Adolescent Medicine* 152, no. 2 (1998): 147–149.

12. S. Fischer, J. Vinall, M. Pavlova, et al., "Role of Anxiety in Young Children's Pain Memory Development after Surgery," *Pain* 160, no. 4 (2019): 965–972; M. Noel, M. Pavlova, T. Lund, et al., "The Role of Narrative in the Development of Children's Pain Memories: Influences of Father- and Mother-Child Reminiscing on Children's Recall of Pain," *Pain* 160, no. 8 (2019): 1866–1875.

13. J. A. Rabbitts, E. Fisher, B. N. Rosenbloom, and T. M. Palermo, "Prevalence and Predictors of Chronic Postsurgical Pain in Children: A Systematic Review and Meta-Analysis," *Journal of Pain* 18, no. 6 (2017): 605–614.

14. K. P. Chua, C. M. Harbaugh, C. M. Brummett, et al., "Association of Perioperative Opioid Prescriptions with Risk of Complications after

Tonsillectomy in Children," *JAMA Otolaryngology—Head and Neck Surgery* 145, no. 10 (2019): 911–918.

15. L. I. Kelley-Quon, M. G. Kirkpatrick, R. L. Ricca, et al., "Guidelines for Opioid Prescribing in Children and Adolescents after Surgery: An Expert Panel Opinion," *JAMA Surgery* 156, no. 1 (2021): 76–90.

16. S. J. Friedrichsdorf and L. Goubert, "Pediatric Pain Treatment and Prevention for Hospitalized Children," *Pain Reports* 5, no. 1 (2020), e804; R. B. Mitchell, S. M. Archer, S. L. Ishman, et al., "Clinical Practice Guideline: Tonsillectomy in Children (Update)—Executive Summary," *Otolaryngology—Head and Neck Surgery* 160, no. 2 (2019): 187–205.

17. B. N. Rosenbloom, M. G. Pagé, L. Isaac, et al., "Pediatric Chronic Postsurgical Pain and Functional Disability: A Prospective Study of Risk Factors up to One Year after Major Surgery," *Journal of Pain Research* 12 (2019): 3079–3098.

18. B. Dagg, P. Forgeron, G. Macartney, and J. Chartrand, "Adolescent Patients' Management of Postoperative Pain after Discharge: A Qualitative Study," *Pain Management Nursing* 21, no. 6 (2020): 565–571.

19. B. A. Krauss and B. S. Krauss, "Managing the Frightened Child," *Annals of Emergency Medicine* 74, no. 1 (2019): 30–35; B. S. Krauss, B. A. Krauss, and S. M. Green, "Managing Procedural Anxiety in Children," *New England Journal of Medicine* 374, no. 16 (2016), e19.

Chapter 6: My Tummy Hurts

1. J. J. Korterink, K. Diederen, M. A. Benninga, and M. M. Tabbers, "Epidemiology of Pediatric Functional Abdominal Pain Disorders: A Meta-Analysis," *PLoS One* 10, no. 5 (2015), e0126982.

2. Korterink et al., "Epidemiology of Pediatric Functional Abdominal Pain Disorders."

3. L. S. Walker, T. A. Lipani, J. W. Greene, et al., "Recurrent Abdominal Pain: Symptom Subtypes Based on the Rome II Criteria for Pediatric Functional Gastrointestinal Disorders," *Journal of Pediatric Gastroenterology and Nutrition* 38, no. 2 (2004): 187–191.

4. J. S. Matthews, "Recurrent Abdominal Pain in Children," *Ulster Medical Journal* 7, no. 3 (1938): 179–206.

5. J. Apley and N. Naish, "Recurrent Abdominal Pains: A Field Survey of 1,000 School Children," *Archives of Disease in Childhood* 33, no. 168 (1958): 165–170.

6. M. Green, "Diagnosis and Treatment: Psychogenic, Recurrent, Abdominal Pain," *Pediatrics* 40, no. 1 (1967): 84–89; D. G. Marshall, "Diagnosis and Treatment: Recurrent Abdominal Pain in Children: A Surgeon's Viewpoint," *Pediatrics* 40, no. 6 (1967): 1024–1026.

7. Green, "Diagnosis and Treatment."

8. M. Saps, C. Blank, S. Khan, et al., "Seasonal Variation in the Presentation of Abdominal Pain," *Journal of Pediatric Gastroenterology and Nutrition* 46, no. 3 (2008): 279–284; M. Saps, S. Hudgens, R. Mody, K. Lasch, V. Harikrishnan, and C. Baum, "Seasonal Patterns of Abdominal Pain Consultations among Adults and Children," *Journal of Pediatric Gastroenterology and Nutrition* 56, no. 3 (2013): 290–296; T. V. Schrijver, P. L. Brand, and J. Bekhof, "Seasonal Variation of Diseases in Children: A 6-Year Prospective Cohort Study in a General Hospital," *European Journal of Pediatrics* 175, no. 4 (2016): 457–464.

9. Saps et al., "Seasonal Variation."

10. C. Q. Chen, J. Fichna, M. Bashashati, Y. Y. Li, and M. Storr, "Distribution, Function and Physiological Role of Melatonin in the Lower Gut," *World Journal of Gastroenterology* 17, no. 34 (2011): 3888–3898.

11. A. Abbasnezhad, R. Amani, E. Hajiani, P. Alavinejad, B. Cheraghian, and A. Ghadiri, "Effect of Vitamin D on Gastrointestinal Symptoms and Health-Related Quality of Life in Irritable Bowel Syndrome Patients: A Randomized Double-Blind Clinical Trial," *Neurogastroenterology and Motility* 28, no. 10 (2016): 1533–1544.

12. K. Hanevik, K. A. Wensaas, G. Rortveit, G. E. Eide, K. Morch, and N. Langeland, "Irritable Bowel Syndrome and Chronic Fatigue 6 Years after Giardia Infection: A Controlled Prospective Cohort Study," *Clinical Infectious Diseases* 59, no. 10 (2014): 1394–1400; K. A. Wensaas, K. Hanevik, T. Hausken, et al., "Postinfectious and Sporadic Functional Gastrointestinal Disorders Have Different Prevalences and Rates of Overlap: Results from a Controlled Cohort Study 3 Years after Acute Giardiasis," *Neurogastroenterology and Motility* 28, no. 10 (2016): 1561–1569.

13. L. Pensabene, V. Talarico, D. Concolino, et al., "Postinfectious Functional Gastrointestinal Disorders in Children: A Multicenter

Prospective Study," *Journal of Pediatrics* 166, no. 4 (2015): 903–907. e901.

14. E. Coss-Adame and S. S. Rao, "Brain and Gut Interactions in Irritable Bowel Syndrome: New Paradigms and New Understandings," *Current Gastroenterology Reports* 16, no. 4 (2014): article 379.

15. C. Ibeakanma, F. Ochoa-Cortes, M. Miranda-Morales, et al., "Brain-Gut Interactions Increase Peripheral Nociceptive Signaling in Mice with Postinfectious Irritable Bowel Syndrome," *Gastroenterology* 141, no. 6 (2011): 2098–2108.e2095; I. Spreadbury, F. Ochoa-Cortes, C. Ibeakanma, N. Martin, D. Hurlbut, and S. J. Vanner, "Concurrent Psychological Stress and Infectious Colitis Is Key to Sustaining Enhanced Peripheral Sensory Signaling," *Neurogastroenterology and Motility* 27, no. 3 (2015): 347–355.

16. M. C. Morris, L. S. Walker, S. Bruehl, A. L. Stone, A. S. Mielock, and U. Rao, "Impaired Conditioned Pain Modulation in Youth with Functional Abdominal Pain," *Pain* 157, no. 10 (2016): 2375–2381.

17. L. M. Dufton, M. J. Dunn, L. S. Slosky, B. E. Compas, "Self-Reported and Laboratory-Based Responses to Stress in Children with Recurrent Pain and Anxiety," *Journal of Pediatric Psychology* 36, no. 1 (2011): 95–105.

18. S. E. Williams, C. A. Smith, S. P. Bruehl, J. Gigante, and L. S. Walker, "Medical Evaluation of Children with Chronic Abdominal Pain: Impact of Diagnosis, Physician Practice Orientation, and Maternal Trait Anxiety on Mothers' Responses to the Evaluation," *Pain* 146, no. 3 (2009): 283–292.

19. A. A. Shah, C. K. Zogg, S. N. Zafar, et al., "Analgesic Access for Acute Abdominal Pain in the Emergency Department among Racial/Ethnic Minority Patients: A Nationwide Examination," *Medical Care* 53, no. 12 (2015): 1000–1009; M. Ghoshal, H. Shapiro, K. Todd, and M. E. Schatman, "Chronic Noncancer Pain Management and Systemic Racism: Time to Move toward Equal Care Standards," *Journal of Pain Research* 13 (2020): 2825–2836.

20. G. D. Shelby, K. C. Shirkey, A. L. Sherman, et al., "Functional Abdominal Pain in Childhood and Long-Term Vulnerability to Anxiety Disorders," *Pediatrics* 132, no. 3 (2013): 475–482.

21. D. K. Chitkara, M. A. L. van Tilburg, N. Blois-Martin, and W. E. Whitehead, "Early Life Risk Factors That Contribute to Irritable

Bowel Syndrome in Adults: A Systematic Review," *American Journal of Gastroenterology* 103, no. 3 (2008): 765–774.

22. R. A. Abbott, A. E. Martin, T. V. Newlove-Delgado, et al., "Psychosocial Interventions for Recurrent Abdominal Pain in Childhood," *Cochrane Database of Systematic Reviews,* January 10, 2017, CD010971; S. M. van der Veek, B. H. Derkx, M. A. Benninga, F. Boer, and E. de Haan, "Cognitive Behavior Therapy for Pediatric Functional Abdominal Pain: A Randomized Controlled Trial," *Pediatrics* 132, no. 5 (2013), e1163–1172.

23. A. Chmielewska and H. Szajewska, "Systematic Review of Randomised Controlled Trials: Probiotics for Functional Constipation," *World Journal of Gastroenterology* 16, no. 1 (2010): 69–75; F. C. L. Ding, M. Karkhaneh, L. Zorzela, H. Jou, and S. Vohra, "Probiotics for Paediatric Functional Abdominal Pain Disorders: A Rapid Review," *Paediatrics and Child Health* 24, no. 6 (2019): 383–394; C. A. M. Wegh, M. A. Benninga, and M. M. Tabbers, "Effectiveness of Probiotics in Children with Functional Abdominal Pain Disorders and Functional Constipation: A Systematic Review," *Journal of Clinical Gastroenterology* 52 suppl. 1 (2018), Proceedings from the 9th Probiotics, Prebiotics and New Foods Meeting, Rome, September 2017, S10–S26.

Chapter 7: When The Pain *Is* In Your Head

1. S. Taheri, "Effect of Exclusion of Frequently Consumed Dietary Triggers in a Cohort of Children with Chronic Primary Headache," *Nutrition and Health* 23, no. 1 (2017): 47–50.

2. J. G. Millichap and M. M. Yee, "The Diet Factor in Pediatric and Adolescent Migraine," *Pediatric Neurology* 28, no. 1 (2003): 9–15.

3. I. Abu-Arafeh, S. Razak, B. Sivaraman, and C. Graham, "Prevalence of Headache and Migraine in Children and Adolescents: A Systematic Review of Population-Based Studies," *Developmental Medicine and Child Neurology* 52, no. 12 (2010): 1088–1097; I. Abu-Arefeh and G. Russell, "Prevalence of Headache and Migraine in Schoolchildren," *BMJ* 309, no. 6957 (1994): 765–769; E. Conicella, U. Raucci, N. Vanacore, et al., "The Child with Headache in a Pediatric Emergency Department," *Headache* 48, no. 7 (2008): 1005–1011; T. M. Lateef, K. R. Merikangas, J. He, et al., "Headache in a National Sample of

American Children: Prevalence and Comorbidity," *Journal of Child Neurology* 24, no. 5 (2009): 536–543; H. Rhee, "Prevalence and Predictors of Headaches in US Adolescents," *Headache: The Journal of Head and Face Pain* 40, no. 7 (2000): 528–538; R. Rossi, A. Versace, B. Lauria, et al., "Headache in the Pediatric Emergency Department: A 5-Year Retrospective Study," *Cephalalgia* 38, no. 11 (2018): 1765–1772; C. Wober-Bingol, "Epidemiology of Migraine and Headache in Children and Adolescents," *Current Pain and Headache Reports* 17, no. 6 (2013), article 341; H. Rhee, M. S. Miles, C. T. Halpern, and D. Holditch-Davis, "Prevalence of Recurrent Physical Symptoms in U.S. Adolescents," *Pediatric Nursing* 31, no. 4 (2005): 314–319, 350.

4. Wober-Bingol, "Epidemiology of Migraine and Headache"; H. Rhee, "Relationships between Physical Symptoms and Pubertal Development," *Journal of Pediatric Health Care* 19, no. 2 (2005): 95–103.

5. D. Borsook, N. Maleki, L. Becerra, and B. McEwen, "Understanding Migraine through the Lens of Maladaptive Stress Responses: A Model Disease of Allostatic Load," *Neuron* 73, no. 2 (2012): 219–234.

6. D. G. Finniss, T. J. Kaptchuk, F. Miller, and F. Benedetti, "Biological, Clinical, and Ethical Advances of Placebo Effects," *Lancet* 375, no. 9715 (2010): 686–695; J. Marchant, "Placebos: Honest Fakery," *Nature* 535, no. 7611 (2016): S14–S15.

7. S. W. Powers, C. S. Coffey, L. A. Chamberlin, et al., "Trial of Amitriptyline, Topiramate, and Placebo for Pediatric Migraine," *New England Journal of Medicine* 376, no. 2 (2017): 115–124.

8. S. Cormier, G. L. Lavigne, M. Choinière, and P. Rainville, "Expectations Predict Chronic Pain Treatment Outcomes," *Pain* 157, no. 2 (2016): 329–338; A. Esparham, A. Herbert, E. Pierzchalski, et al., "Pediatric Headache Clinic Model: Implementation of Integrative Therapies in Practice," *Children* 5, no. 6 (2018), article 74; V. Faria, C. Linnman, A. Lebel, and D. Borsook, "Harnessing the Placebo Effect in Pediatric Migraine Clinic," *Journal of Pediatrics* 165, no. 4 (2014): 659–665.

9. S. Ballou, A. Beath, T. J. Kaptchuk, et al., "Factors Associated with Response to Placebo in Patients with Irritable Bowel Syndrome and Constipation," *Clinical Gastroenterology and Hepatology* 16, no. 11

(2018): 1738–1744.e1731; F. Benedetti, E. Carlino, and A. Pollo, "How Placebos Change the Patient's Brain," *Neuropsychopharmacology* 36, no. 1 (2011): 339–354; T. J. Kaptchuk and F. G. Miller, "Open Label Placebo: Can Honestly Prescribed Placebos Evoke Meaningful Therapeutic Benefits? *BMJ* 363 (2018), k3889.

10. Esparham et al., "Pediatric Headache Clinic Model."

Chapter 8: Too Much Pain, No Gain

1. D. R. Patel, A. Yamasaki, and K. Brown, "Epidemiology of Sports-Related Musculoskeletal Injuries in Young Athletes in United States," *Translational Pediatrics* 6, no. 3 (2017): 160–166.

2. N. A. Smith, T. Chounthirath, and H. Xiang, "Soccer-Related Injuries Treated in Emergency Departments: 1990–2014," *Pediatrics* 138, no. 4 (2016), e20160346.

3. E. R. Dodwell, L. E. Lamont, D. W. Green, T. J. Pan, R. G. Marx, and S. Lyman, "20 Years of Pediatric Anterior Cruciate Ligament Reconstruction in New York State," *American Journal of Sports Medicine* 42, no. 3 (2014): 675–680.

4. R. Hall, K. Barber Foss, T. E. Hewett, and G. D. Myer, "Sport Specialization's Association with an Increased Risk of Developing Anterior Knee Pain in Adolescent Female Athletes," *Journal of Sport Rehabilitation* 24, no. 1 (2015): 31–35; T. Junge, L. Runge, B. Juul-Kristensen, and N. Wedderkopp, "Risk Factors for Knee Injuries in Children 8 to 15 Years: The CHAMPS Study DK," *Medicine and Science in Sports and Exercise* 48, no. 4 (2016): 655–662.

5. "The Female ACL: Why Is It More Prone to Injury?" editorial, *Journal of Orthopaedics* 13, no. 2 (2016): A1–A4.

6. J. L. Hodgins, M. Vitale, R. R. Arons, and C. S Ahmad, "Epidemiology of Medial Ulnar Collateral Ligament Reconstruction: A 10-Year Study in New York State," *American Journal of Sports Medicine* 44, no. 3 (2016): 729–734.

7. Hall et al., "Sport Specialization's Association"; Junge et al., "Risk Factors for Knee Injuries"; L. Babcock, C. S. Olsen, D. M. Jaffe, and J. C. Leonard, "Cervical Spine Injuries in Children Associated with Sports and Recreational Activities," *Pediatric Emergency Care* 34, no. 10 (2018): 677–686; K. D. Barber Foss, G. D. Myer, and T. E. Hewett, "Epidemiology of Basketball, Soccer, and Volleyball

Injuries in Middle-School Female Athletes," *Physician and Sportsmedicine* 42, no. 2 (2014): 146–153; J. de Inocencio, M. A. Carro, M. Flores, C. Carpio, S. Mesa, and M. Marin, "Epidemiology of Musculoskeletal Pain in a Pediatric Emergency Department," *Rheumatology International* 36, no. 1 (2016): 83–89; I. Dizdarevic, M. Bishop, N. Sgromolo, S. Hammoud, and A. Atanda Jr., "Approach to the Pediatric Athlete with Back Pain: More Than Just the Pars," *Physician and Sportsmedicine* 43, no. 4 (2015): 421–431; M. H. Guddal, S. O. Stensland, M. C. Smastuen, M. B. Johnsen, J. A. Zwart, and K. Storheim, "Physical Activity Level and Sport Participation in Relation to Musculoskeletal Pain in a Population-Based Study of Adolescents: The Young-HUNT Study," *Orthopaedic Journal of Sports Medicine* 5, no. 1 (2017), 2325967116685543; M. R. Guerra, J. R. Estelles, Y. A. Abdouni, D. F. Falcochio, J. R. Rosa, and L. H. Catani, "Frequency of Wrist Growth Plate Injury in Young Gymnasts at a Training Center," *Acta Ortopedica Brasileira* 24, no. 4 (2016): 204–207; E. Jespersen, R. Holst, C. Franz, C. T. Rexen, H. Klakk, and N. Wedderkopp, "Overuse and Traumatic Extremity Injuries in Schoolchildren Surveyed with Weekly Text Messages over 2.5 Years," *Scandinavian Journal of Medicine and Science in Sports* 24, no. 5 (2014): 807–813; M. Noll, E. A. Silveira, and I. S. Avelar, "Evaluation of Factors Associated with Severe and Frequent Back Pain in High School Athletes," *PloS One* 12, no. 2 (2017), e0171978; A. Stracciolini, R. Casciano, H. Levey Friedman, C. J. Stein, W. P. Meehan 3rd, and L. J. Micheli, "Pediatric Sports Injuries: A Comparison of Males versus Females," *American Journal of Sports Medicine* 42, no. 4 (2014): 965–972; J. S. Yang, J. G. Stepan, L. Dvoracek, R. W. Wright, R. H. Brophy, and M. V. Smith, "Fast-Pitch Softball Pitchers Experience a Significant Increase in Pain and Fatigue during a Single High School Season," *HSS Journal: The Musculoskeletal Journal of Hospital for Special Surgery* 12, no. 2 (2016): 111–118; A. X. Yin, D. Sugimoto, D. J. Martin, and A. Stracciolini, "Pediatric Dance Injuries: A Cross-Sectional Epidemiological Study," *PM and R: The Journal of Injury, Function, and Rehabilitation* 8, no. 4 (2016): 348–355.

8. M. A. Bryan, A. Rowhani-Rahbar, R. D. Comstock, and F. Rivara, "Sports- and Recreation-Related Concussions in US Youth," *Pediatrics* 138, no. 1 (2016), e20154635; V. G. Coronado, T. Haileyesus,

T. A. Cheng, et al., "Trends in Sports- and Recreation-Related Traumatic Brain Injuries Treated in US Emergency Departments: The National Electronic Injury Surveillance System-All Injury Program (NEISS-AIP) 2001–2012," *Journal of Head Trauma Rehabilitation* 30, no. 3 (2015): 185–197; T. Pfister, K. Pfister, B. Hagel, W. A. Ghali, and P. E. Ronksley, "The Incidence of Concussion in Youth Sports: A Systematic Review and Meta-analysis," *British Journal of Sports Medicine* 50, no. 5 (2016): 292–297; J. A. Rosenthal, R. E. Foraker, C. L. Collins, and R. D. Comstock, "National High School Athlete Concussion Rates from 2005–2006 to 2011–2012," *American Journal of Sports Medicine* 42, no. 7 (2014): 1710–1715.

9. M. P. Ithurburn, M. V. Paterno, K. R. Ford, T. E. Hewett, and L. C. Schmitt, "Young Athletes after Anterior Cruciate Ligament Reconstruction with Single-Leg Landing Asymmetries at the Time of Return to Sport Demonstrate Decreased Knee Function 2 Years Later," *American Journal of Sports Medicine* 45, no. 11 (2017): 2604–2613; J. L. Whittaker, L. J. Woodhouse, A. Nettel-Aguirre, and C. A. Emery, "Outcomes Associated with Early Post-traumatic Osteoarthritis and Other Negative Health Consequences 3–10 Years Following Knee Joint Injury in Youth Sport," *Osteoarthritis and Cartilage* 23, no. 7 (2015): 1122–1129.

10. A. L. Holley, A. C. Wilson, and T. M. Palermo, "Predictors of the Transition from Acute to Persistent Musculoskeletal Pain in Children and Adolescents: A Prospective Study," *Pain* 158, no. 5 (2017): 794–801.

11. K. Grimmer and M. Williams, "Gender-Age Environmental Associates of Adolescent Low Back Pain," *Applied Ergonomics* 31, no. 4 (2000): 343–360.

12. T. I. Nilsen, A. Holtermann, and P. J. Mork, "Physical Exercise, Body Mass Index, and Risk of Chronic Pain in the Low Back and Neck/Shoulders: Longitudinal Data from the Nord-Trondelag Health Study," *American Journal of Epidemiology* 174, no. 3 (2011): 267–273.

13. G. S. Roebuck, D. M. Urquhart, L. Knox, et al., "Psychological Factors Associated with Ultramarathon Runners' Supranormal Pain Tolerance: A Pilot Study," *Journal of Pain* 19, no. 12 (2018): 1406–1415; J. Tesarz, A. Gerhardt, K. Schommer, R. D. Treede, and W. Eich, "Alterations in Endogenous Pain Modulation in Endurance Athletes:

An Experimental Study Using Quantitative Sensory Testing and the Cold-Pressor Task," *Pain* 154, no. 7 (2013): 1022–1029.

14. G. L. Fanucchi, A. Stewart, R. Jordaan, and P. Becker, "Exercise Reduces the Intensity and Prevalence of Low Back Pain in 12–13 Year Old Children: A Randomised Trial," *Australian Journal of Physiotherapy* 55, no. 2 (2009): 97–104; J. Tesarz, A. K. Schuster, M. Hartmann, A. Gerhardt, and W. Eich, "Pain Perception in Athletes Compared to Normally Active Controls: A Systematic Review with Meta-analysis," *Pain* 153, no. 6 (2012): 1253–1262; M. Geisler, L. Eichelkraut, W. H. R. Miltner, and T. Weiss, "Expectation of Exercise in Trained Athletes Results In a Reduction of Central Processing to Nociceptive Stimulation," *Behavioural Brain Research* 356 (2019): 314–321.

15. R. J. Elbin, A. Sufrinko, P. Schatz, et al., "Removal from Play after Concussion and Recovery Time," *Pediatrics* 138, no. 3 (2016), e20160910.

16. D. G. Thomas, J. N. Apps, R. G. Hoffmann, M. McCrea, and T. Hammeke, "Benefits of Strict Rest after Acute Concussion: A Randomized Controlled Trial," *Pediatrics* 135, no. 2 (2015): 213–223.

17. W. Mittenberg, G. Tremont, R. E. Zielinski, S. Fichera, and K. R. Rayls, "Cognitive-behavioral Prevention of Postconcussion Syndrome," *Archives of Clinical Neuropsychology* 11, no. 2 (1996): 139–145.

18. C. A. McCarty, D, Zatzick, E. Stein, J. Wang, R. Hilt, and F. P. Rivara, "Collaborative Care for Adolescents with Persistent Postconcussive Symptoms: A Randomized Trial," *Pediatrics* 138, no. 4 (2016), e20160459.

19. D. J. Thomas, K. Coxe, H. Li, et al., "Length of Recovery from Sports-Related Concussions in Pediatric Patients Treated at Concussion Clinics," *Clinical Journal of Sport Medicine* 28, no. 1 (2018): 56–63.

Chapter 9: Pain as a Disease State

1. S. Bruehl, "Complex Regional Pain Syndrome," *BMJ* 351 (2015): h2730.

2. E. Krane, "The Mystery of Chronic Pain," TED talk, May 19, 2011, https://www.youtube.com/watch?v=J6—CMhcCfQ.

3. L. W. Crock and M. T. Baldridge, "A Role for the Microbiota in Complex Regional Pain Syndrome?" *Neurobiology of Pain* 8 (2020), https://www.sciencedirect.com/science/article/pii/S2452073X2030012X; E. S. Haight, T. E. Forman, S. A. Cordonnier, et al., "Microglial Modulation as a Target for Chronic Pain: From the Bench to the Bedside and Back," *Anesthesia and Analgesia* 128, no. 4 (April 2019): 737–746, doi: 10.1213/ANE.0000000000004033.

4. A. M. de Rooij, M. de Mos, J. J. van Hilten, et al., "Increased Risk of Complex Regional Pain Syndrome in Siblings of Patients?" *Journal of Pain* 10, no. 12 (2009): 1250–1255; D. E. van Rooijen, D. L. Roelen, W. Verduijn, et al., "Genetic HLA Associations in Complex Regional Pain Syndrome with and without Dystonia," *Journal of Pain* 13, no. 8 (2012): 784–789.

5. D. D. Sherry, C. A. Wallace, C. Kelley, M. Kidder, and L. Sapp, "Short- and Long-Term Outcomes of Children with Complex Regional Pain Syndrome Type I Treated with Exercise Therapy," *Clinical Journal of Pain* 15, no. 3 (1999): 218–223; R. Weissmann and Y. Uziel, "Pediatric Complex Regional Pain Syndrome: A Review," *Pediatric Rheumatology Online Journal* 14, no. 1 (2016): 29; R. Wilder, C. B. Berde, M. Wolohan, M. Vieyra, B. Masek, and I. Micheli, "Reflex Sympathetic Dystrophy in Children: Clinical Characteristics and Follow Up of Seventy Patients," *Journal of Bone and Joint Surgery, American Volume* 74, no. 6 (1992): 910–919.

6. D. D. Sherry and R. Weisman, "Psychologic Aspects of Childhood Reflex Neurovascular Dystrophy," *Pediatrics* 81, no. 4 (1988): 572–578; J. Wager, H. Brehmer, G. Hirschfeld, and B. Zernikow, "Psychological Distress and Stressful Life Events in Pediatric Complex Regional Pain Syndrome," *Pain Research and Management* 20, no. 4 (2015): 189–194.

7. J. Marinus, G. L. Moseley, F. Birklein, et al., "Clinical Features and Pathophysiology of Complex Regional Pain Syndrome," *Lancet Neurology* 10, no. 7 (2011): 637–648.

8. A. J. Terkelsen, F. W. Bach, and T. S. Jensen, "Experimental Forearm Immobilization in Humans Induces Cold and Mechanical Hyperalgesia," *Anesthesiology* 109, no. 2 (2008): 297–307.

9. S. Butler, M. Nyman, and T. Gordh, "Immobility in Volunteers Transiently Produces Signs and Symptoms of Complex Regional Pain Syndrome," in *Proceedings of the 9th World Congress on Pain,* 657–660 (Seattle: IASP Press, 2000).

10. N. Erpelding, L. Simons, A. Lebel, et al., "Rapid Treatment-Induced Brain Changes in Pediatric CRPS," *Brain Structure and Function* 221, no. 2 (2016): 1095–1111; L. E. Simons, M. Pielech, N. Erpelding, et al., "The Responsive Amygdala: Treatment-Induced Alterations in Functional Connectivity in Pediatric Complex Regional Pain Syndrome," *Pain* 155, no. 9 (2014): 1727–1742.

11. Sherry et al., "Short- and Long-Term Outcomes"; V. Brooke and S. Janselewitz, "Outcomes of Children with Complex Regional Pain Syndrome after Intensive Inpatient Rehabilitation," *PM and R* 4, no. 5 (2012): 349–354; Y. Takahashi, T. Tominaga, K. Okawa, K. Tanaka, "Recovery from Acute Pediatric Complex Regional Pain Syndrome Type I after Ankle Sprain by Early Pharmacological and Physical Therapies in Primary Care: A Case Report," *Journal of Pain Research* 11 (2018): 2859–2866.

12. S. Kashikar-Zuck, C. King, T. V. Ting, and L. M. Arnold, "Juvenile Fibromyalgia: Different from the Adult Chronic Pain Syndrome?" *Current Rheumatology Reports* 18, no. 4 (2016): 19; S. Kashikar-Zuck, T. V. Ting, L. M. Arnold, et al., "Cognitive Behavioral Therapy for the Treatment of Juvenile Fibromyalgia: A Multisite, Single-Blind, Randomized, Controlled Clinical Trial," *Arthritis and Rheumatism* 64, no. 1 (2012): 297–305.

13. Kashikar-Zuck et al., "Juvenile Fibromyalgia": Kashikar-Zuck et al., "Cognitive Behavioral Therapy."

14. S. Sil, S. Thomas, C. DiCesare, et al., "Preliminary Evidence of Altered Biomechanics in Adolescents with Juvenile Fibromyalgia," *Arthritis Care and Research* 67, no. 1 (2015): 102–111; S. T. Tran, S. Thomas S, C. DiCesare, et al., "A Pilot Study of Biomechanical Assessment before and after an Integrative Training Program for Adolescents with Juvenile Fibromyalgia," *Pediatric Rheumatology Online Journal* 14, no. 1 (2016): 43.

15. Tran et al., "Pilot Study of Biomechanical Assessment"; S. Kashikar-Zuck, W. R. Black, M. Pfeiffer, et al., "Pilot Randomized Trial of Integrated Cognitive-Behavioral Therapy and Neuromuscular Training for Juvenile Fibromyalgia: The FIT Teens Program,"

Journal of Pain 19, no. 9 (2018): 1049–1062; S. Kashikar-Zuck, S. T. Tran, K. Barnett, et al., "A Qualitative Examination of a New Combined Cognitive-Behavioral and Neuromuscular Training Intervention for Juvenile Fibromyalgia," *Clinical Journal of Pain* 32, no. 1 (2016): 70–81.

16. Kashikar-Zuck et al., "Pilot Randomized Trial of Integrated Cognitive-Behavioral Therapy"; Kashikar-Zuck et al., "Qualitative Examination of a New Combined Cognitive-Behavioral and Neuromuscular Training."

17. S. Kashikar-Zuck, N. Cunningham, J. Peugh, et al., "Long-Term Outcomes of Adolescents with Juvenile-Onset Fibromyalgia into Adulthood and Impact of Depressive Symptoms on Functioning over Time," *Pain* 160, no. 2 (2019): 433–441; S. Kashikar-Zuck, N. Cunningham, S. Sil, et al., "Long-Term Outcomes of Adolescents with Juvenile-Onset Fibromyalgia in Early Adulthood," *Pediatrics* 133, no. 3 (2014): e592–600.

Chapter 10: More than Just Medication

1. T. M. Palermo, M. Slack, C. Zhou, R. Aaron, E. Fisher, and S. Rodriguez, "Waiting for a Pediatric Chronic Pain Clinic Evaluation: A Prospective Study Characterizing Waiting Times and Symptom Trajectories," *Journal of Pain* 20, no. 3 (2019): 339–347.

2. "Pediatric Pain Clinics 2021," Special Interest Group on Pain in Childhood, International Association for the Study of Pain, n.d., accessed November 26, 2021, http://childpain.org/wp-content /uploads/2021/01/Pediatric-Chronic-Pain-Programs-2021-Update .pdf.

3. T. Hechler, M. Kanstrup, A. L. Holley, et al., "Systematic Review on Intensive Interdisciplinary Pain Treatment of Children with Chronic Pain," *Pediatrics* 136, no. 1 (2015): 115–127; G. Revivo, D. K. Amstutz, C. M. Gagnon, and Z. L. McCormick, "Interdisciplinary Pain Management Improves Pain and Function in Pediatric Patients with Chronic Pain Associated with Joint Hypermobility Syndrome," *P M and R* 11, no. 2 (2019): 150–157; L. E. Simons, D. E. Logan, L. Chastain, and M. Cerullo, "Engagement in Multidisciplinary Interventions for Pediatric Chronic Pain: Parental Expectations, Barriers, and Child Outcomes," *Clinical Journal of Pain* 26, no. 4

(2010): 291–299; L. E. Simons, C. B. Sieberg, M. Pielech, C. Conroy, and D. E. Logan, "What Does It Take? Comparing Intensive Rehabilitation to Outpatient Treatment for Children with Significant Pain-Related Disability," *Journal of Pediatric Psychology* 38, no. 2 (2013): 213–223; H. Tick, A. Nielsen, K. R. Pelletier, et al., "Evidence-Based Nonpharmacologic Strategies for Comprehensive Pain Care: The Consortium Pain Task Force White Paper," *Explore* 14, no. 3 (2018): 177–211.

4. L. S. Walker, A. L. Stone, G. T. Han, et al., "Internet-Delivered Cognitive Behavioral Therapy for Youth with Functional Abdominal Pain: A Randomized Clinical Trial Testing Differential Efficacy by Patient Subgroup," *Pain* 162, no. 12 (2021): 2945–2955.

5. Hechler et al., "Systematic Review on Intensive Interdisciplinary Pain Treatment"; Simons et al., "What Does It Take?"

6. Revivo et al., "Interdisciplinary Pain Management"; H. Robins, V. Perron, L. C. Heathcote, and L. E. Simons, "Pain Neuroscience Education: State of the Art and Application in Pediatrics," *Children* 3, no. 4 (2016): 43.

7. E. Fisher, E. Law, J. Dudeney, T. M. Palermo, G. Stewart, and C. Eccleston, "Psychological Therapies for the Management of Chronic and Recurrent Pain in Children and Adolescents," *Cochrane Database of Systematic Reviews*, October 1, 2018, CD003968.

8. Revivo et al., "Interdisciplinary Pain Management."

9. The acronym GET stands for graded in vivo exposure treatment, a method that has helped adults with chronic pain. For more on this program evaluating its efficacy with youthful patients, see L. E. Simons, J. W. S. Vlaeyen, L. Declercq, et al., "Avoid or Engage? Outcomes of Graded Exposure in Youth with Chronic Pain Using a Sequential Replicated Single-Case Randomized Design," *Pain* 161, no. 3 (2020): 520–531.

10. N. E. Mahrer, J. I. Gold, M. Luu, and P. M. Herman, "A Cost-Analysis of an Interdisciplinary Pediatric Chronic Pain Clinic," *Journal of Pain* 19, no. 2 (2018): 158–165.

11. Tick et al., "Evidence-Based Nonpharmacologic Strategies"; A. A. Wren, A. C. Ross, G. D'Souza, et al., "Multidisciplinary Pain Management for Pediatric Patients with Acute and Chronic Pain: A Foundational Treatment Approach When Prescribing Opioids," *Children* 6, no. 2 (2019): 33.

12. L. I. Kelley-Quon, M. G. Kirkpatrick, R. L. Ricca, et al., "Guidelines for Opioid Prescribing in Children and Adolescents after Surgery: An Expert Panel Opinion," *JAMA Surgery* 156, no. 1 (2021): 76–90; N. L. Schechter and G. A. Walco, "The Potential Impact on Children of the CDC Guideline for Prescribing Opioids for Chronic Pain: Above All, Do No Harm," *JAMA Pediatrics* 170, no. 5 (2016): 425–426.

13. R. A. Moore and H. J. McQuay, "Prevalence of Opioid Adverse Events in Chronic Non-malignant Pain: Systematic Review of Randomised Trials of Oral Opioids," *Arthritis Research and Therapy* 7, no. 5 (2005): R1046–1051.

14. J. R. Gaither, V. Shabanova, and J. M. Leventhal, "US National Trends in Pediatric Deaths from Prescription and Illicit Opioids, 1999–2016," *JAMA Network Open* 1, no. 8 (2018), e186558.

15. E. M. Raney, H. J. P. van Bosse, K. G. Shea, J. M. Abzug, and R. M. Schwend, "Current State of the Opioid Epidemic as It Pertains to Pediatric Orthopaedics from the Advocacy Committee of the Pediatric Orthopaedic Society of North America," *Journal of Pediatric Orthopedics* 38, no. 5 (2018): e238–e244.

16. E. T. Chow, J. D. Otis, and L. E. Simons, "The Longitudinal Impact of Parent Distress and Behavior on Functional Outcomes among Youth with Chronic Pain," *Journal of Pain* 17, no. 6 (2016): 729–738.

17. L. Caes, T. Vervoort, C. Eccleston, M. Vandenhende, and L. Goubert, "Parental Catastrophizing about Child's Pain and Its Relationship with Activity Restriction: The Mediating Role of Parental Distress," *Pain* 152, no. 1 (2011): 212–222; L. Caes, T. Vervoort, Z. Trost, and L. Goubert, "Impact of Parental Catastrophizing and Contextual Threat on Parents' Emotional and Behavioral Responses to Their Child's Pain," *Pain* 153, no. 3 (2012): 687–695; L. S. Walker, S. E. Williams, C. A. Smith, J. Garber, D. A. Van Slyke, and T. A. Lipani, "Parent Attention versus Distraction: Impact on Symptom Complaints by Children with and without Chronic Functional Abdominal Pain," *Pain* 122, no. 1–2 (2006): 43–52.

18. Simons et al., "Engagement in Multidisciplinary Interventions."

19. T. M. Palermo, A. C. Wilson, M. Peters, A. Lewandowski, and H. Somhegyi, "Randomized Controlled Trial of an Internet-Delivered Family Cognitive-Behavioral Therapy Intervention for Children and Adolescents with Chronic Pain," *Pain* 146, no. 1 (2009): 205–213.

20. A. C. Long and T. M. Palermo, "Web-Based Management of Adolescent Chronic Pain: Development and Usability Testing of an Online Family Cognitive Behavioral Therapy Program," *Journal of Pediatric Psychology* 34, no. 5 (2009): 511–516.

21. E. Fisher, E. Law, J. Dudeney, C. Eccleston, and T. M. Palermo, "Psychological Therapies (Remotely Delivered) for the Management of Chronic and Recurrent Pain in Children and Adolescents," *Cochrane Database of Systematic Reviews,* April 2, 2019, CD011118.

22. R. Eijlers, E. M. W. J. Utens, L. M. Staals, et al., "Systematic Review and Meta-analysis of Virtual Reality in Pediatrics: Effects on Pain and Anxiety," *Anesthesia and Analgesia* 129, no. 5 (2019): 1344–1353; A. S. Won, J. Bailey, J. Bailenson, C. Tataru, I. A. Yoon, and B. Golianu, "Immersive Virtual Reality for Pediatric Pain," *Children* 4, no. 7 (2017): 52.

23. R. Coakley, T. Wihak, J. Kossowsky, C. Iversen, and C. Donado, "The Comfort Ability Pain Management Workshop: A Preliminary, Nonrandomized Investigation of a Brief, Cognitive, Biobehavioral, and Parent Training Intervention for Pediatric Chronic Pain," *Journal of Pediatric Psychology* 43, no. 3 (2018): 252–265.

Chapter 11: Family Ties

1. M. A. Clementi, P. Faraji, K. Poppert Cordts, et al., "Parent Factors Are Associated with Pain and Activity Limitations in Youth with Acute Musculoskeletal Pain: A Cohort Study," *Clinical Journal of Pain* 35, no. 3 (2019): 222–228.

2. T. M. Palermo, C. R. Valrie, and C. W. Karlson, "Family and Parent Influences on Pediatric Chronic Pain: A Developmental Perspective," *American Psychologist* 69, no. 2 (2014): 142–152.

3. C. T. Chambers, K. D. Craig, and S. M. Bennett, "The Impact of Maternal Behavior on Children's Pain Experiences: An Experimental Analysis," *Journal of Pediatric Psychology* 27, no. 3 (2002): 293–301; L. S. Walker, S. E. Williams, C. A. Smith, J. Garber, D. A. Van Slyke, and T. A. Lipani, "Parent Attention versus Distraction: Impact on Symptom Complaints by Children with and without Chronic Functional Abdominal Pain," *Pain* 122, no. 1–2 (2006): 43–52.

4. J. W. Guite, R. L. McCue, J. L. Sherker, D. D. Sherry, and J. B. Rose, "Relationships among Pain, Protective Parental Responses, and Disability for Adolescents with Chronic Musculoskeletal Pain: The Mediating Role of Pain Catastrophizing," *Clinical Journal of Pain* 27, no. 9 (2011): 775–781; A. M. Lynch-Jordan, S. Kashikar-Zuck, A. Szabova, and K. R. Goldschneider, "The Interplay of Parent and Adolescent Catastrophizing and Its Impact on Adolescents' Pain, Functioning, and Pain Behavior," *Clinical Journal of Pain* 29, no. 8 (2013): 681–688.

5. A. Bandura, *Social Learning Theory* (Englewood Cliffs, NJ: Prentice-Hall, 1977).

6. A. C. Wilson, A. Moss, T. M. Palermo, and J. L. Fales, "Parent Pain and Catastrophizing Are Associated with Pain, Somatic Symptoms, and Pain-Related Disability among Early Adolescents," *Journal of Pediatric Psychology* 39, no. 4 (2014): 418–426.

7. A. C. Wilson and J. L. Fales, "Parenting in the Context of Chronic Pain: A Controlled Study of Parents with Chronic Pain," *Clinical Journal of Pain* 31, no. 8 (2015): 689–698.

8. Wilson and Fales, "Parenting in the Context of Chronic Pain."

9. A. C. Wilson, A. L. Holley, A. Stone, J. L. Fales, and T. M. Palermo, "Pain, Physical, and Psychosocial Functioning in Adolescents at Risk for Developing Chronic Pain: A Longitudinal Case-Control Study," *Journal of Pain* 21, no. 3–4 (2020): 418–429.

10. S. Krokstad, A. Langhammer, K. Hveem, et al., "Cohort Profile: The HUNT Study, Norway," *International Journal of Epidemiology* 42, no. 4 (2013): 968–977.

11. G. B. Hoftun, P. R. Romundstad, and M. Rygg, "Association of Parental Chronic Pain with Chronic Pain in the Adolescent and Young Adult: Family Linkage Data from the HUNT Study," *JAMA Pediatrics* 167, no. 1 (2013): 61–69.

12. J. Dahlhamer, J. Lucas, C. Zelaya, et al., "Prevalence of Chronic Pain and High-Impact Chronic Pain among Adults—United States, 2016," *MMWR Morbidity and Mortality Weekly Report* 67, no. 36 (2018): 1001–1006.

13. K. S. Higgins, K. A. Birnie, C. T. Chambers, et al., "Offspring of Parents with Chronic Pain: A Systematic Review and Meta-analysis of Pain, Health, Psychological, and Family Outcomes," *Pain* 156, no. 11 (2015): 2256–2266.

14. W. Umberger, D. Martsolf, A. Jacobson, J. Risko, M. Patterson, and M. Calabro, "The Shroud: Ways Adolescents Manage Living with Parental Chronic Pain," *Journal of Nursing Scholarship* 45, no. 4 (2013): 344–354.

15. Higgins et al., "Offspring of Parents with Chronic Pain."

16. A. L. Stone, A. L. Holley, N. F. Dieckmann, and A. C. Wilson, "Use of the PROMIS-29(R) to Identify Subgroups of Mothers with Chronic Pain," *Health Psychology* 38, no. 5 (2019): 422–430; A. C. Wilson, A. L. Stone, K. L. Poppert Cordts, et al., "Baseline Characteristics of a Dyadic Cohort of Mothers with Chronic Pain and Their Children," *Clinical Journal of Pain* 36, no. 10 (2020): 782–792.

17. K. S. Higgins, C. T. Chambers, N. O. Rosen, et al., "Testing the Intergenerational Model of Transmission of Risk for Chronic Pain from Parents to Their Children: An Empirical Investigation of Social Transmission Pathways," *Pain* 160, no. 11 (2019): 2544–2553; A. L. Stone, S. Bruehl, C. A. Smith, J. Garber, and L. S. Walker, "Social Learning Pathways in the Relation between Parental Chronic Pain and Daily Pain Severity and Functional Impairment in Adolescents with Functional Abdominal Pain," *Pain* 159, no. 2 (2018): 298–305; E. Van Lierde, L. Goubert, T. Vervoort, G. Hughes, and E. Van den Bussche, "Learning to Fear Pain after Observing Another's Pain: An Experimental Study in Schoolchildren," *European Journal of Pain* 24, no. 4 (2020): 791–806.

18. B. D. Darnall, J. A. Sturgeon, M.-C. Kao, J. M. Hah, and S. C. Mackey, "From Catastrophizing to Recovery: A Pilot Study of a Single-Session Treatment for Pain Catastrophizing," *Journal of Pain Research* 7 (2014): 219–226.

19. Chambers et al., "The Impact of Maternal Behavior"; K. E. Boerner, C. T. Chambers, P. J. McGrath, V. LoLordo, and R. Uher, "The Effect of Parental Modeling on Child Pain Responses: The Role of Parent and Child Sex," *Journal of Pain* 18, no. 6 (2017): 702–715.

Chapter 12: The Invisible Burden of Pain

1. E. Igler, A. Lang, K. Balistreri, E. Sejkora, A. Drendel, and W. H. Davies, "Parents Reliably Identify Pain Dismissal by Pediatric Providers," *Clinical Journal of Pain* 36, no. 2 (2020): 80–87.

2. V. L. Shavers, A. Bakos, and V. B. Sheppard, "Race, Ethnicity, and Pain among the US Adult Population," *Journal of Health Care for the Poor and Underserved* 21, no. 1 (2010): 177–220; R. C. Tait and J. T. Chibnall, "Racial/Ethnic Disparities in the Assessment and Treatment of Pain: Psychosocial Perspectives," *American Psychologist* 69, no. 2 (2014): 131–141.

3. Igler et al., "Parents Reliably Identify Pain Dismissal."

4. E. O. Wakefield, W. T. Zempsky, R. M. Puhl, and M. D. Litt, "Conceptualizing Pain-Related Stigma in Adolescent Chronic Pain: A Literature Review and Preliminary Focus Group Findings," *Pain Reports* 3, suppl. 1 (2018), e679.

5. K. Hamberg, G. Risberg, E. E. Johansson, and G. Westman, "Gender Bias in Physicians' Management of Neck Pain: A Study of the Answers in a Swedish National Examination," *Journal of Women's Health and Gender-Based Medicine* 11, no. 7 (2002): 653–666.

6. A. Samulowitz, I. Gremyr, E. Eriksson, and G. Hensing, "'Brave Men' and 'Emotional Women': A Theory-Guided Literature Review on Gender Bias in Health Care and Gendered Norms towards Patients with Chronic Pain," *Pain Research and Management* 2018 (2018), 6358624.

7. A. T. Hirsh, N. A. Hollingshead, M. S. Matthias, M. J. Bair, and K. Kroenke, "The Influence of Patient Sex, Provider Sex, and Sexist Attitudes on Pain Treatment Decisions," *Journal of Pain* 15, no. 5 (2014): 551–559; B. D. Earp, J. T. Monrad, M. LaFrance, J. A. Bargh, L. L. Cohen, and J. A. Richeson, "Gender Bias in Pediatric Pain Assessment," *Journal of Pediatric Psychology* 44, no. 4 (2019): 403–414; L. L. Cohen, J. Cobb, and S. R. Martin, "Gender Biases in Adult Ratings of Pediatric Pain," *Children's Health Care* 43, no. 2 (2014): 87–95.

8. K. C. Johnson, A. J. LeBlanc, J. Deardorff, and W. O. Bockting, "Invalidation Experiences among Non-binary Adolescents," *Journal of Sex Research* 57, no. 2 (2020): 222–233; G. N. Rider, B. J. McMorris, A. L. Gower, E. Coleman, and M. E. Eisenberg, "Health and Care Utilization of Transgender and Gender Nonconforming Youth: A Population-Based Study," *Pediatrics* 141, no. 3 (2018), e20171683.

9. J. D. Greenspan, R. M. Craft, L. LeResche, et al., "Studying Sex and Gender Differences in Pain and Analgesia: A Consensus Report," *Pain* 132 (2007): S26–S45.

10. Agency for Healthcare Research and Quality, "Chartbook on Health Care for Blacks," Part 2: "Trends in Priorities of the Heckler Report," AHRQ, Rockville, MD, 2016, last reviewed June 2018, accessed June 29, 2020, https://www.ahrq.gov/research/findings/nhqrdr /chartbooks/blackhealth/part2.html; K. P. Chua, C. M. Harbaugh, C. M. Brummett, et al., "Association of Perioperative Opioid Prescriptions with Risk of Complications after Tonsillectomy in Children," *JAMA Otolaryngology Head Neck Surgery* 145, no. 10 (2019): 911–918.

11. US Department of Health and Human Services, "Report of the Secretary's Task Force on Black and Minority Health" (Washington, DC: US Government Printing Office, 1985), 1219–1222.

12. T. J. Cunningham, J. B. Croft, Y. Liu, H. Lu, P. I. Eke, and W. H. Giles, "Vital Signs: Racial Disparities in Age-Specific Mortality among Blacks or African Americans—United States, 1999–2015," *MMWR Morbidity and Mortality Weekly Report* 66, no. 17 (2017): 444.

13. Shavers et al., "Race, Ethnicity, and Pain"; P. Lee, M. Le Saux, R. Siegel, et al., "Racial and Ethnic Disparities in the Management of Acute Pain in US Emergency Departments: Meta-analysis and Systematic Review," *American Journal of Emergency Medicine* 37, no. 9 (2019): 1770–1777; R. Wyatt, "Pain and Ethnicity," *AMA Journal of Ethics* 15, no. 5 (2013): 449–454; T. M. Anastas, M. M. Miller, N. A. Hollingshead, J. C. Stewart, K. L. Rand, and A. T. Hirsh, "The Unique and Interactive Effects of Patient Race, Patient Socioeconomic Status, and Provider Attitudes on Chronic Pain Care Decisions," *Annals of Behavioral Medicine* 54, no. 10 (2020): 771–782.

14. C. S. Cleeland, R. Gonin, L. Baez, P. Loehrer, and K. J. Pandya, "Pain and Treatment of Pain in Minority Patients with Cancer: The Eastern Cooperative Oncology Group Minority Outpatient Pain Study," *Annals of Internal Medicine* 127, no. 9 (1997): 813–816; H. P. Freeman and R. Payne, "Racial Injustice in Health Care," *New England Journal of Medicine* 342, no. 14 (2000): 1045–1047; J. A. Sabin and A. G. Greenwald, "The Influence of Implicit Bias on Treatment Recommendations for 4 Common Pediatric Conditions: Pain, Urinary Tract Infection, Attention Deficit Hyperactivity Disorder, and Asthma," *American Journal of Public Health* 102, no. 5 (2012): 988–995; M. M. Miller, A. E. Williams, T. C. B. Zapolski, K. L. Rand,

and A. T. Hirsh, "Assessment and Treatment Recommendations for Pediatric Pain: The Influence of Patient Race, Patient Gender, and Provider Pain-Related Attitudes," *Journal of Pain* 21, no. 1–2 (2020): 225–237.

15. M. K. Goyal, N. Kuppermann, S. D, Cleary, S. J. Teach, and J. M. Chamberlain, "Racial Disparities in Pain Management of Children with Appendicitis in Emergency Departments," *JAMA Pediatrics* 169, no. 11 (2015): 996–1002.

16. M. K. Goyal, T. J. Johnson, J. M. Chamberlain, et al., "Racial and Ethnic Differences in Emergency Department Pain Management of Children with Fractures," *Pediatrics* 145, no. 5 (2020): e20193370.

17. K. M. Hoffman, S. Trawalter, J. R. Axt, and M. N. Oliver, "Racial Bias in Pain Assessment and Treatment Recommendations, and False Beliefs about Biological Differences between Blacks and Whites," *Proceedings of the National Academy of Sciences* 113, no. 16 (2016): 4296–4301.

18. E. van Schaik, A. Howson, and J. Sabin, "Healthcare Disparities" course, MedEdPortal, *Journal of Teaching and Learning Resources,* Association of American Medical Colleges, 2014, https://www.mededportal.org/doi/full/10.15766/mep_2374-8265.9675.

19. J. A. Sabin, "How We Fail Black Patients in Pain," Association of American Medical Colleges, January 6, 2020, https://www.aamc.org/news-insights/how-we-fail-black-patients-pain.

20. Project Implicit, Implicit Association Test, n.d., https://implicit.harvard.edu/implicit/education.html.

21. White Coats for Black Lives, https://whitecoats4blacklives.org/about/.

22. D. Bulgin, P. Tanabe, and C. Jenerette, "Stigma of Sickle Cell Disease: A Systematic Review," *Issues in Mental Health Nursing* 39, no. 8 (2018): 675–686; D. P. R. Burnes, B. J. Antle, C. C. Williams, and L. Cook, "Mothers Raising Children with Sickle Cell Disease at the Intersection of Race, Gender, and Illness Stigma," *Health and Social Work* 33, no. 3 (2008): 211–220; E. O. Wakefield, J. M. Popp, L. P. Dale, J. P. Santanelli, A. Pantaleao, and W. T. Zempsky, "Perceived Racial Bias and Health-Related Stigma among Youth with Sickle Cell Disease," *Journal of Developmental Behavior and Pediatrics* 38, no. 2 (2017): 129–134.

23. Burnes et al., "Mothers Raising Children with Sickle Cell Disease."

24. C. B. Groenewald, M. Giles, and T. M. Palermo, "School Absence Associated with Childhood Pain in the United States," *Clinical Journal of Pain* 35, no. 6 (2019): 525–531.

25. D. E. Logan, L. E. Simons, and K. J. Kaczynski, "School Functioning in Adolescents with Chronic Pain: The Role of Depressive Symptoms in School Impairment," *Journal of Pediatric Psychology* 34, no. 8 (2009): 882–892.

26. N. N. Youssef, T. G. Murphy, S. Schuckalo, C. Intile, and J. Rosh, "School Nurse Knowledge and Perceptions of Recurrent Abdominal Pain: Opportunity for Therapeutic Alliance?" *Clinical Pediatrics* 46, no. 4 (2007): 340–344.

27. D. E. Logan, S. P. Catanese, R. M. Coakley, and L. Scharff, "Chronic Pain in the Classroom: Teachers' Attributions about the Causes of Chronic Pain," *Journal of School Health* 77, no. 5 (2007): 248–256.

28. P. A. Forgeron, S. King, J. N. Stinson, P. J. McGrath, A. J. MacDonald, and C. T. Chambers, "Social Functioning and Peer Relationships in Children and Adolescents with Chronic Pain: A Systematic Review," *Pain Research and Management* 15, no. 1 (2010): 27–41.

29. Logan et al., "School Functioning in Adolescents with Chronic Pain"; L. E. Simons, D. E. Logan, L. Chastain, and M. Stein, "The Relation of Social Functioning to School Impairment among Adolescents with Chronic Pain," *Clinical Journal of Pain* 26, no. 1 (2010): 16–22.

30. V. La Buissonniere-Ariza, D. Hart, S. C. Schneider, et al., "Quality and Correlates of Peer Relationships in Youths with Chronic Pain," *Child Psychiatry and Human Development* 49, no. 6 (2018): 865–874.

31. J. V. Campo, J. Bridge, M. Ehmann, et al., "Recurrent Abdominal Pain, Anxiety, and Depression in Primary Care," *Pediatrics* 113, no. 4 (2004): 817–824; S. Kashikar-Zuck, K. R. Goldschneider, S. W. Powers, M. H. Vaught, and A. D. Hershey, "Depression and Functional Disability in Chronic Pediatric Pain," *Clinical Journal of Pain* 17, no. 4 (2001): 341–349; M. H. Bromberg, E. F. Law, and T. M. Palermo, "Suicidal Ideation in Adolescents with and without Chronic Pain," *Clinical Journal of Pain* 33, no. 1 (2017): 21–27;

M. A. L. van Tilburg, N. J. Spence, W. E. Whitehead, S. Bangdiwala, and D. B. Goldston, "Chronic Pain in Adolescents Is Associated with Suicidal Thoughts and Behaviors," *Journal of Pain* 12, no. 10 (2011): 1032–1039.

32. D. E. Logan, R. L. Claar, J. W. Guite, et al., "Factor Structure of the Children's Depression Inventory in a Multisite Sample of Children and Adolescents with Chronic Pain," *Journal of Pain* 14, no. 7 (2013): 689–698.

33. G. J. G. Asmundson and J. Katz, "Understanding the Co-occurrence of Anxiety Disorders and Chronic Pain: State-of-the-Art," *Depression and Anxiety* 26, no. 10 (2009): 888–901.

34. M. Tegethoff, A. Belardi, E. Stalujanis, and G. Meinlschmidt, "Comorbidity of Mental Disorders and Chronic Pain: Chronology of Onset in Adolescents of a National Representative Cohort," *Journal of Pain* 16, no. 10 (2015): 1054–1064.

35. A. M. McIntosh, L. S. Hall, Y. Zeng, et al., "Genetic and Environmental Risk for Chronic Pain and the Contribution of Risk Variants for Major Depressive Disorder: A Family-Based Mixed-Model Analysis." *PLoS Medicine* 13, no. 8 (2016), e1002090; W. Meng, M. J. Adams, P. Reel, et al., "Genetic Correlations between Pain Phenotypes and Depression and Neuroticism," *European Journal of Human Genetics* 28, no. 3 (2020): 358–366.

36. A. Riggenbach, L. Goubert, S. Van Petegem, and R. Amouroux, "Basic Psychological Needs in Adolescents with Chronic Pain: A Self-Determination Perspective," *Pain Research and Management* 2019 (2019), 8629581.

Acknowledgments

This book could not have been written without the generous participation of our sources. To the researchers, clinicians, and most of all, to the families who shared their expertise, experiences, and lives with us: we are forever indebted to you.

To Laurie Fox, our agent, you have been our steadfast guiding light throughout this entire publishing process. We thank you from the bottom of our hearts for believing in us and this book, and for your tenacity, warmth, and wit.

To Andrew Kinney, our editor, thank you for seeing the potential in this book and for your editing along the way. We are also grateful for the entire team at Harvard University Press.

Beyond the people who deserve our joint gratitude, there are additional people, special to each of us, we would like to thank.

From Rachel: There are so many wonderful people who have buoyed me in my career and in the writing of this book. I would like to start by thanking my writer friends. To Taffy Brodesser-Akner, Andrea Lynn, and Anya Hoffman: You each helped me jumpstart my freelance career in different, marvelous ways, at a crucial point in my life. Thank you for giving me the courage to pursue the kind of writing assignments and projects I wanted to do. To Kim Brown, Michael Levitin, and Jocelyn Wiener, my inspiring and caring friends and former classmates: Your influence helped shape me into the journalist I am today. To Marcy Paul and Debbie Tola: Thank you for "getting it" and for always being able to offer a supportive shoulder and thoughtful insight. To my colleagues at Consumer Reports: I am ever grateful for your support, smarts, and friendship.

I must also give a heartfelt thank you to all of my dear friends and extended family who asked about the book and believed in me.

A special thank you goes to Emily Wakefield and her team at Connecticut Children's Medical Center, for making it possible for me to attend their Comfort Ability workshop.

To my brother and sister-in-law, David and Judi Rabkin: I don't know where I'd be without your love, advice, and cheerleading.

To my parents, Eric and Elizabeth Rabkin: Your unconditional love has shaped my entire life. Dad: Thank you for your astute editing of this book, your wise counsel, and for being my first and best writing teacher. Mom: Thank you for always being there for me, for talking me through life's challenges, and for championing me with endless enthusiasm.

Lenn and Annika: I love you more than you will ever know. Thank you for being the strong, sweet, and loving people you are.

Russ: You made this book possible. Thank you for taking care of the kids while I was working late nights and weekends; thank you for your smart edits to this book; and most of all, thank you for your humor, patience, calm, and love.

Anna: Thank you for reaching out to me all those years ago and asking me to collaborate. I am honored that you trusted me to tell this important story with you. Your expertise, research savvy, and sunny attitude have been invaluable.

From Anna: This book was nurtured into existence by an incredibly supportive community of colleagues and friends over the course of many years, and inspired by the lived experiences of patients with pain who I have had the privilege of working with.

I first want to thank Dr. Tonya Palermo, my postdoctoral mentor, who first introduced me to pediatric pain as a research field. Tonya: Your commitment to helping children with pain and their families, and to conducting meaningful clinical research continues to inspire me to do my own best work.

My first introduction to the pediatric pain community was through the Pain in Child Health (PICH) training program, which enriched my understanding of pain and my connections to colleagues from around the world. My gratitude goes to Drs. Patrick McGrath and Allen Finley for founding this important program, and for all of the faculty and trainees I have had the joy of getting to know over the years.

I would also like to thank all of my pediatric pain and psychology colleagues at Oregon Health & Science University and beyond, especially Dr. Amy Holley, who is the best office mate, collaborator, and friend I could ever hope to work with.

To my parents, Philip and Mary Long: Thank you for your unending love and support for me and for my educational aspirations. And thank you for modeling and teaching enthusiasm about learning, love and kindness for others, and a sense of wonder and awe about the natural world.

Cora, Conrad, and Camille: You are the best children a mom could ask for. Thank you for making our family fun and joyful, and for always letting me know when I have been at my computer for far too long. I love you three.

Daniel: It is impossible to work alongside you (literally during Covid times) and not catch a little of the writing bug. Thank you for generously sharing your edits, your literary agent, and your years of writing experience. And thank you for supporting all the extra time that this project took.

Rachel: This book would not have happened without you! Thank you for writing about your own lived experience with pain, being willing to take this leap with me, and for all of your hard work and patience with the process.

Index